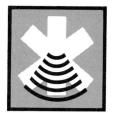

Ultrasound
In
Emergency
Medicine

Michael Heller, MD, FACEP
Clinical Professor of Medicine
Temple University School of Medicine
Philadelphia, Pennsylvania
Program Director
Emergency Medicine Residency
   of the Lehigh Valley
Bethlehem, Pennsylvania

Dietrich Jehle, MD, FACEP
Director of Emergency Services
Erie County Medical Center
Associate Professor and Vice Chairman
Department of Emergency Medicine
State University of New York at Buffalo
School of Medicine
Buffalo, New York

W.B. SAUNDERS COMPANY
A Division of Harcourt Brace & Company
Philadelphia • London • Toronto • Montreal • Sydney • Tokyo

W.B. SAUNDERS COMPANY
A Division of Harcourt Brace & Company

The Curtis Center
Independence Square West
Philadelphia, Pennsylvania 19106

Library of Congress Cataloging-in-Publication Data

Heller, Michael.
    Ultrasound in emergency medicine / Michael Heller, Dietrich Jehle.
—1st ed.
        p. cm.
    ISBN 0–7216–4506–2
    1. Diagnosis, Ultrasonic. 2. Emergency medicine. 3. Medical emergencies
—Diagnosis. I. Jehle, Dietrich. II. Title.
    [DNLM: 1. Ultrasonography. 2. Emergencies. 3. Emergency Medicine—
instrumentation. 4. Emergency Medicine—education. WB 289 H477u 1995]
RC78.7.U4H45 1995
616.07'543—dc20
DNLM/DLC   94-13906

ULTRASOUND IN EMERGENCY MEDICINE   ISBN 0–7216–4506–2

Last digit is the print number: 9 8 7 6 5 4 3 2

Contributors

Mark E. Deutchman, MD, FAAFP
Associate Professor of Family Medicine, University of Colorado,
Denver, Colorado; Formerly Associate Professor of Family Medicine, University
of Tennessee, Memphis, Tennessee

David Plummer, MD, FACEP
Senior Associate Physician, Department of Emergency Medicine, Hennepin
County Medical Center, Minneapolis, Minnesota

Foreword

In September 1979, Emergency Medicine was formally recognized as the 23rd discipline to receive specialty recognition by the American Board of Medical Specialties. Such recognition solidified the concept that a unique body of knowledge was the province of emergency medicine and that a unique specialist, the emergency physician, was a fully recognized addition to the practice of clinical medicine and surgery. During subsequent years, the specialty has continued to focus on its primary mission, the ability to recognize immediately and respond appropriately to acute clinical conditions. Such a clinical focus has led increasingly to bedside evaluation with point-of-service testing carried out in the emergency center. Perhaps no such modality is as useful a tool to facilitate this as is the imaging provided through bedside ultrasound. The future portends — and may well demand — an exponential increase in ambulatory activities to provide diagnostic and observational services formerly occurring within a specialized inpatient setting and under the purview of a traditional, inpatient-oriented, specialist. With the blurring of once-rigid specialty boundaries, progressive emergency centers and emergency physicians have already expanded their roles to encompass new responsibilities. Both technological improvements and economic developments have provided additional impetus; improvement in image quality, portability, and affordability occur with each new generation of diagnostic equipment. At the same time, fundamental changes in health care delivery and reimbursement have enhanced the value of rapid, cost-effective diagnostic strategies such as emergency ultrasound. The authors, recognizing this trend, have become the leaders from the discipline of emergency medicine in exploring and developing the appropriate utilization of ultrasound within the emergency center. Their research and experience has been translated into this premier and utterly unique text, which serves to provide the practicing emergency physician with a prudent and pragmatic approach to the use of emergency ultrasound.

Now is a momentous time for our specialty, and this text's emergence is most propitious. It provides fundamental information that will be essential to every exemplar emergency physician's professional database. Additionally, it will be an invaluable text for the graduate training programs, which seek to provide the next generation of emergency physicians with instruction and experience in the use of bedside ultrasound. The time is precisely right. The text is exceptionally focused. And the authors' vision is exceedingly clear. The specialty has a unique opportunity to move forward with its mission of diagnosing and treating acutely ill or injured patients.

DAVID K. WAGNER, MD
Professor and Chairman
Department of Emergency Medicine
Medical College of Pennsylvania

Preface

This textbook has but one purpose: to help emergency medicine residents and practitioners incorporate the use of ultrasound into their clinical practice. The manner in which ultrasound is utilized by our specialty will vary tremendously during the foreseeable future. In some institutions, particularly those with large teaching programs and excellent around-the-clock availability of ultrasound services, the emergency physician's challenge continues to be that of selecting the appropriate patients for sonographic studies and understanding what the results mean in terms of clinical decision-making. Their primary interest in the "hands on" aspects is driven by the desire to teach (as emergency medicine faculty) and learn (as emergency medicine residents). This book is designed for those physicians precisely. At the opposite extreme are physicians working in an environment where traditional ultrasound services are delayed or absent for much of the time. These physicians need to perform many of their own ultrasound examinations and interpret the results on a fairly routine basis. For these physicians, ultrasound is simply another clinical skill that must be mastered to provide their patients with the best possible care. This book was written for these physicians also. Finally, there are likely many more emergency physicians who practice in hospitals where traditional ultrasound specialists are often but not always available and the need to perform ultrasound studies at the bedside occurs less regularly, but at times with great urgency. This book is written for those physicians most of all.

We have no illusions as to the permanence of this work. Both the specialty of emergency medicine and the applications of ultrasound are evolving too rapidly, and the very environment in which we and all physicians work is changing even faster. What we can hope for is that this text will provide a framework for the use of ultrasound in our specialty and that this framework will survive long after medical and technological changes prompt revisions in the content.

The framework is based on the premise that ultrasound has become so important to modern emergency medicine practice that some of our patients literally cannot live without it. It is necessary therefore to develop the means by which immediate availability of selected ultrasound studies is a reality. At the same time, we must recognize the limitations of time, skill, and equipment that dictate that we use each of these to optimal benefit.

The structure of the text is organized to reflect our conservatism with regard to emergency ultrasound. Only six major ultrasound uses are regarded as primary emergency department applications for ultrasound. Four of these (abdominal aortic aneurysm, traumatic hemoperitoneum, ectopic pregnancy, and pericardial tamponade) are acutely life-threatening emergencies for which delay cannot be justified. The other two (acute gallbladder disease and obstructive uropathy) are included because of their great frequency and their significance in terms of morbidity, and the uncontested efficacy of straightforward scanning techniques in aiding in their diagnosis and clinical decision-making. Several "other" emergency department applications of sonography are reflected in Chapter 3, which emphasizes what information can be expected to be obtained from each particular sonographic study. Not everyone will agree with our selections in each category, but few, we hope, will disagree with our goals.

MICHAEL HELLER, MD
DIETRICH JEHLE, MD

Acknowledgments

A new text represents the work of numerous individuals, each person providing a distinctive contribution to the end product. We are particularly indebted to our contributors, David Plummer, MD, and Mark Deutchman, MD, whose scholarship and formidable work in ultrasonography have helped shape this text. The quality of the final product is a testament to their work.

Two individuals who deserve special recognition for their invaluable contributions as illustrator and photographer are John Nyquist and James Ulrich. John's attention to detail and arduous efforts reflect his paramount dedication to medical illustration. The quality of Jim's photography is a gold standard for all medical photographers to emulate.

The support, patience, and understanding of our families are truly valued. To Mike's wife Diane and son Gregory, and Dietrich's wife Theresa and children Christopher, Zachary and Gabrielle, we owe our deepest appreciation.

We would like also to thank the staff at W.B. Saunders for their contributions. In particular, we need to thank Nellie McGrew, Developmental Editor, and Judy Fletcher, Senior Acquisitions Editor, for their tireless efforts in bringing this text to final publication.

Our secretaries Sherrie Heffernan, Trista Green, and Evelyn Roycroft deserve special mention for their assistance in preparing this manuscript.

Finally, there is a group of dedicated emergency physicians and courageous colleagues in other specialties, including Radiology, Gynecology, Cardiology, Surgery, and Family Practice, who have been instrumental in bringing ultrasound to the bedside in Emergency Medicine. To them we express our gratitude and acknowledge an everlasting debt.

Authors' Note

The reader may have already noted that this text is structured somewhat differently from other texts on emergency imaging procedures. The first chapter is traditional, dealing essentially with nonclinical aspects of ultrasound, presenting the basic knowledge that the emergency physician should acquire to utilize ultrasound and to understand the rest of the book. The bulk of the text, comprising the next two chapters, deals with the clinical aspects of ultrasound studies. These are not arranged by direct anatomic considerations but rather are grouped into primary emergency department studies and "additional" emergency department applications. This was done for two reasons.

Most importantly the classification of a particular indication as either primary or secondary reflects our judgment as practicing emergency physicians utilizing ultrasound as to the potential benefits that immediate bedside ultrasound would have for that condition. Those applications classified as "primary" are judged to have the greatest potential for bedside use by the emergency physician in terms of decreasing morbidity or mortality. Those applications classed as "secondary" or "other" are often legitimate and necessary studies but with significantly less potential for immediately altering the patient's course. The two distinct factors that go into this judgment are the seriousness and time sensitivity of the underlying condition.

The second reason for a given classification is the likelihood that immediate bedside ultrasound would be both helpful and feasible to perform considering the nature of the process and the difficulty of the examination. For example, pericardial tamponade and leaking abdominal aortic aneurysm are two examples of conditions in which time constraints are critical and straightforward scanning techniques may rapidly establish or refute the diagnosis. Acute symptomatic gallbladder disease or acute obstructive uropathy do not bear this same time criticality, but the bedside ultrasound diagnosis of both is likely to be instrumental in guiding further interventions. Acute appendicitis, on the other hand, is listed as a secondary application, not because it is a less serious condition than acute cholecystitis but because the ultrasound examination is difficult and requires a quality of equipment and time that is usually not available in an emergency department setting. As a final example, testicular torsion is a morbid and time-critical event but the (non-Doppler) ultrasound findings are often nonspecific and therefore unlikely to affect the course of the condition. It too merits "secondary" status.

The other reason for organizing the text in this fashion is that as the only emergency medicine ultrasound text it inevitably (and hopefully) will be used by some almost as a handbook, as a quick clinical guide to answer particular questions that develop in the course of practice. By arranging the book according to clinical problems rather than just by particular organs, access to the most appropriate sections can be expedited.

QUESTIONS

It should be emphasized here (and will be repeated later) that an emergency bedside examination, particularly by a nontraditional ultrasound specialist such as an emergency physician, is not equivalent to traditional ultrasound performed in the radiology department. In fact, the two types of examinations are different in terms of time constraints, equipment, goals, and perhaps skill. The emergency department examination is highly focused and in each case needs a yes–no answer to a simple question. These questions can be stated quite simply.

1. Is there evidence of cholecystitis?
2. Is there evidence of obstructive uropathy?
3. Is an abdominal aortic aneurysm present?
4. Is there blood in the abdomen?
5. Is there evidence of a living intrauterine pregnancy?
6. Is there a pericardial effusion?

Clearly the patient who simply has pericardial tamponade ruled out with ultrasound has not undergone a standard echocardiographic examination, just as the patient in whom a normal nontender gallbladder is documented has not undergone a complete hepatobiliary evaluation. It is important that the limited nature of the study be understood by all those involved in the care of the patient, including the patient himself. The medical records should reflect this as well with a notation that states clearly what was and was not seen. For example, the notation "no hydronephrosis, hydroureter or renal calculi seen at bedside ultrasound" is appropriate and accurate; "renal ultrasound within normal limits" is not. The information gained by the emergency department sonogram, like that gained through the stethoscope or anoscope, is one part of a broad clinical picture. Putting those findings in a proper clinical perspective is a major goal of this book.

Contents

CHAPTER 1

Fundamentals

It is not always necessary for clinicians to have a profound understanding of the technologies that they use. One need only consider studies such as impedance plethysmography (IPG), computed tomography (CT), and magnetic resonance imaging (MRI) to appreciate that the intricacies of even commonly used techniques are often poorly understood by the physician. Yet even with these types of examinations, to say nothing of electrocardiograms (ECGs), plain radiography, and radionuclide scanning, the physician who has a basic understanding of the manner in which the information is obtained and displayed is better able to interpret the significance of that information, particularly when complex or unfamiliar results are obtained. This is especially true when diagnostic ultrasound is used for the emergency department patient. In part, this is because diagnostic ultrasound in the symptomatic patient is inherently an interactive technique. Unlike the standard kidney, ureter, and bladder (KUB) examination, for example, which is performed in a standardized manner regardless of the patient's specific complaints or clinical presentation, the ultrasound examination of the abdomen will vary greatly according to the patient's clinical condition, specific complaints, unique anatomy, and symptoms elicited while performing the examination.

When used in this way — as an extension of the emergency physician's clinical examination — ultrasound is clearly the most user-dependent of the imaging techniques. Although standard guidelines and protocols for the performance of ultrasound examinations by the traditional ultrasound specialist and technolo-gist serve as useful guides, the ultrasound examination of the symptomatic emergency patient frequently leads the careful examiner to scan adjacent and even distant regions from the organ that was initially suspected. To accomplish this, nonstandard views are often required, and unfamiliar images that represent normal anatomy, abnormal anatomy, and artifacts are often obtained; as will be explained more fully in the discussion that follows, the physics of ultrasound waves makes production of such artifacts unavoidable. In addition, particular characteristics of the instrumentation used may also lead to artifacts or unusual representations of anatomy; these effects may or may not be avoidable. For all these reasons, a basic understanding of the manner in which ultrasound waves can be used to form images is not merely an intellectual exercise: it has practical, clinical applications.

SOUND AND ULTRASOUND

Most physicians are familiar with some of the characteristics of ordinary sound. Sound waves are transmitted through a medium, such as air, and form a series of compressions and rarefactions. The number of these compressions and rarefactions per second is referred to as frequency and is measured in hertz (Hz); the normal human ear can hear up to about 20,000 Hz. Technically, any frequencies above this range are referred to as ultrasound. Many commercial and military applications of ultrasound have been developed (e.g., submarine detection, jewelry cleaning), but the frequencies found to be of most use for medical imaging are in the range of a few million hertz, expressed in megahertz (MHz). One megahertz equals 10^6 hertz. All the familiar properties of ordinary sound waves, such as their ability to be blocked by a nonconducting medium, transmission, and reflection, apply equally well to ultrasound waves; each of these properties is routinely observed in ultrasound studies.

One way in which ultrasound waves in the megahertz range differ from ordinary sound is in the types of media that transmit them best. For practical purposes, diagnostic medical ultrasound is not transmissible through air or bone, two substances that transmit ordinary sound waves well. Conversely, fluid-containing structures are excellent transmitters of ultrasound waves and, because most of the body's soft tissues are composed largely of water, ultrasound transmission (and therefore, imaging) is eminently feasible. It would be difficult to overstate the importance of these seemingly simple observations. They explain, for example, the relative futility of ultrasound imaging through an air-containing lung or gas-containing loops of bowel or stomach, which will scatter, reflect, or refract most sound waves. It also explains why imaging through bone or gallstones, which reflect or absorb most sound waves, makes visualization of underlying structures impossible. Structures of soft tissue density both transmit and reflect ultrasound waves, allowing one to visualize internal and underlying anatomy. Objects of fluid density transmit sound well; however, sound waves are only reflected from their borders. These effects are schematically illustrated in Figure 1–1.

Unlike standard x-rays, in which a plate sensitive to ionizing radiation is placed distal to the source of the x-ray–producing device, ultrasound images are formed only by those waves that are reflected back toward the source. The urinary bladder shown in Figure 1–2, which transmits most ultrasound waves, produces no image of its internal contents because there are no waves reflected. At the opposite extreme are objects that reflect or absorb all ultrasound waves, as, for example, the gallstone visualized in Figure 1–3. A suitable receiving device could detect the presence and external shape of such an object but could provide no information regarding the object's internal structure because all the waves are reflected or absorbed at the

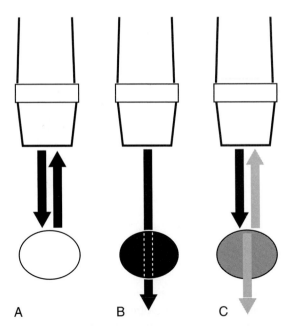

Figure 1–1. *A*, Echogenic image. Ultrasound appearance of a structure that reflects most sound waves. This structure is echogenic or white on the ultrasound screen. *B*, Anechoic image. Ultrasound appearance of a homogeneous structure that transmits sound waves well. This structure is anechoic or dark on the ultrasound screen. It should be noted that most anechoic structures are cystic; however, they may be of solid or soft-tissue density. The posterior echoes usually help define the dark structure: cystic, posterior enhancement; soft tissue/solid, no posterior enhancement. *C*, Gray scale. Imaging of a structure of tissue density that both transmits and reflects ultrasound waves. This structure will appear gray on the ultrasound screen.

object's surface. In either case, poor transmission or complete transmission, useful clinical information might be inferred from the recognition that objects with those particular characteristics are present.

Continuing the analogy with ordinary sound, it should be evident that not only the frequency but also the amplitude of sound and ultrasound waves can vary. Other factors being equal, the intensity of the sound or ultrasound being recorded is greater at greater amplitudes; a device capable of generating a higher amplitude is capable of transmitting that wave further than a device with less energy. For example, sonar devices developed for submarine detection during World War I were of limited power: the amplitude was insufficient to detect deep-running submarines. Sound waves (and light waves as well) also have the property of refraction. That is, the path of the wave bends some-

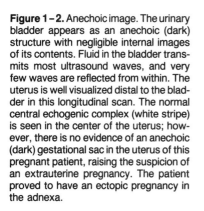

Figure 1–2. Anechoic image. The urinary bladder appears as an anechoic (dark) structure with negligible internal images of its contents. Fluid in the bladder transmits most ultrasound waves, and very few waves are reflected from within. The uterus is well visualized distal to the bladder in this longitudinal scan. The normal central echogenic complex (white stripe) is seen in the center of the uterus; however, there is no evidence of an anechoic (dark) gestational sac in the uterus of this pregnant patient, raising the suspicion of an extrauterine pregnancy. The patient proved to have an ectopic pregnancy in the adnexa.

what as it enters a substance with different conducting speed than the medium through which it was previously transmitted. Figure 1–4 illustrates what happens when a sound (or ultrasound) wave impacts a structure that is sonographically "slower" than the surrounding media. Those waves entering the surface bend slightly to the right within the structure; those being reflected are bent to the left. This leaves a region of relative silence just distal to the edge of the surface. An observer at point X would have difficulty hearing sound waves, and a structure at that point would be difficult to image on ultrasound because there would be relatively fewer incoming waves to be reflected back to the source.

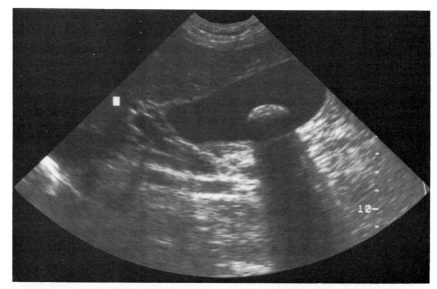

Figure 1–3. Echogenic image. The gallstone in this scan appears as an echogenic (white) structure with dark posterior shadowing. The surface of the gallstone reflects or absorbs all of the ultrasound waves from the transducer. In contrast, the fluid within the gallbladder transmits ultrasound waves well, resulting in its anechoic (dark) appearance.

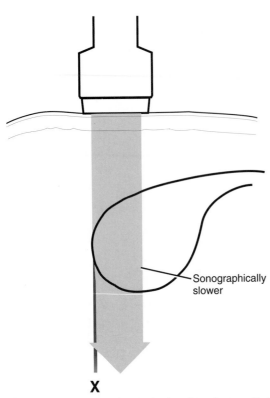

Figure 1–4. Lateral cystic shadowing. Sound waves that pass from a high-velocity medium to a low-velocity medium produce a thin, refractive shadow from the edge of the low-velocity medium. A narrow microphone at X would not receive sound waves and a structure would not image well.

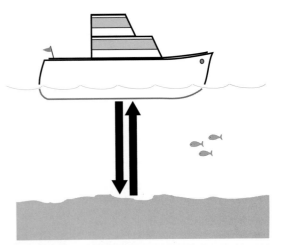

Figure 1–5. A-mode. A single ultrasound signal is transmitted by the ship, reflected off the surface of the ocean floor and returned to the ship. This basic type of imaging corresponds to some of the earliest ultrasound machines, which employed A-mode (amplitude) scanning.

ULTRASOUND PICTURES

Several important qualities of ultrasound images are directly related to the fact that ultrasound devices record only reflected ultrasound waves. Given that the speed of ultrasound transmission through a given medium is constant (which it is), it should be evident that the distance from the ultrasound source to the object is directly related to the time required for the reflected wave to return to that source. If the outgoing and incoming ultrasound signal sent by the surface ship in Figure 1–5 is detected and converted to an audible ping in the headphones of the sonar technician, the depth of the ocean floor would be readily apparent simply by multiplying the time for each returning echo by the speed of sound in water and dividing by two (remember, a sound wave makes a two-way trip). The depth of a submarine can be determined in a similar manner. The same information can be easily displayed graphically. By moving the surface ship, additional soundings

could be taken and an image, as shown in Figure 1–6, could be developed, thus better illustrating the relative position of the ship and the characteristics of the ocean floor. If the surface ship captain invested in a more sophisticated device—capable of generating a rapid series of echoes on a wide path, as illustrated in Figure 1–7A—and displayed the results on an oscilloscope, a representation such as the one shown in Figure 1–7B could be rapidly produced without moving the boat. A corresponding medical example, using a rapid series of echoes along a linear path, is illustrated in Figure 1–8. Finally, with some experience, the sonar technician would notice that not all images on the screen appear equal. Two submarines could be distinguished as being not only at different depths, but as being of different size and perhaps of different shape, as shown in Figure 1–9. In addition, the whale in Figure 1–10A would be noted to be of the same size and depth as the submarine in Figure 1–10B, but the reflecting echo would be less distinct. The sonar technician could logically deduce that ship metal was more highly reflective than whale flesh, and this would help the captain direct depth charges to the appropriate target.

Finally, with the conclusion of hostilities, the captain and the sonar technician might well decide to find commercial applications for their sonographic skills. With equipment of higher frequency and better amplitude and a sonar de-

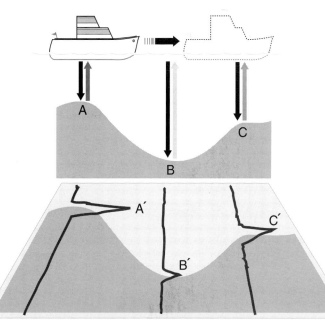

Figure 1-6. Compound B-mode. The ship can be moved across the surface and sound waves transmitted and received at multiple points along the ship's path. The image produced is a summation of many individual signals and is called a compound scan. In A-mode (amplitude mode) imaging, the height of the deflection is related to the intensity of the return sound waves. With B-mode (brightness mode) imaging, this "blip" is converted into a dot on the screen of the ultrasound display. The location of this dot is a function of the time for the sound wave to return to the transducer (vertical axis) and the position of the transducer (horizontal axis), whereas the intensity of this dot is related to the strength of the reflected sound wave. In order to produce a smooth image, the ultrasound machine uses time-gain compensation to take into consideration the attenuation of the ultrasound image as it travels a longer distance. The shaded image displayed represents a compound B-mode scan similar to what was produced with static B-scanners used in the early 1970s.

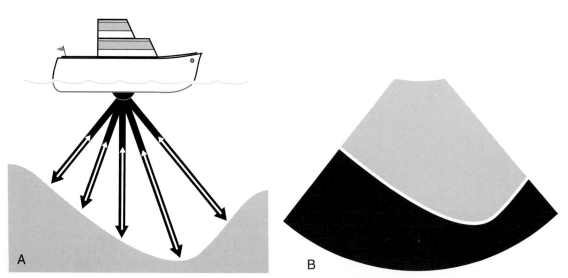

Figure 1-7. A, Real-time B-mode sector scan. This can be produced without moving the ship if the transducer generates a rapid series of echoes on a wide path. The scan can be generated by either mechanically moving the transducer along an arc or electronically firing a series of crystals sequentially to produce a series of ultrasound waves similar to that produced by the mechanical device. B, Real-time B-mode sector scan. Demonstrates the image that is produced on the oscilloscope screen by the sector scanner. Note that some ultrasound waves are transmitted through and some are reflected from the murky water under the ship, which produces a gray image. The surface of the ocean floor strongly reflects sound waves, which produces a bright white border. The sound waves are all absorbed or reflected from the surface of the ocean, resulting in the posterior black shadowing distal to the ocean floor.

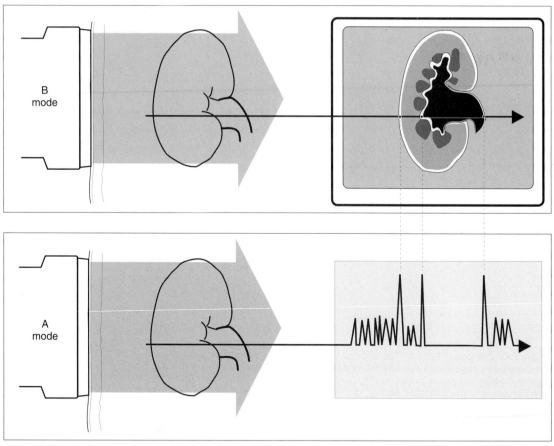

Figure 1–8. A-mode versus B-mode. A rapid series of echoes that are transmitted along a linear path similar to what is seen with a linear array scanner. This diagram demonstrates the appearance of sound waves transmitted and returned to a single piezoelectric crystal in both A-mode (*bottom*) and B-mode (*top*).

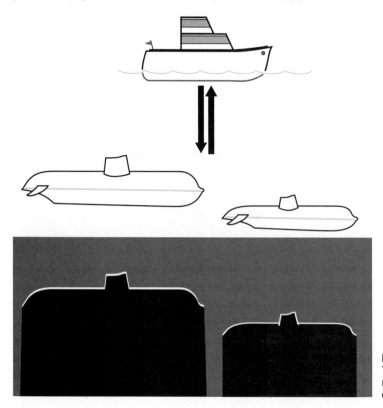

Figure 1–9. Various depths and sizes. The ultrasound appearance of two submarines at different depths and of different sizes.

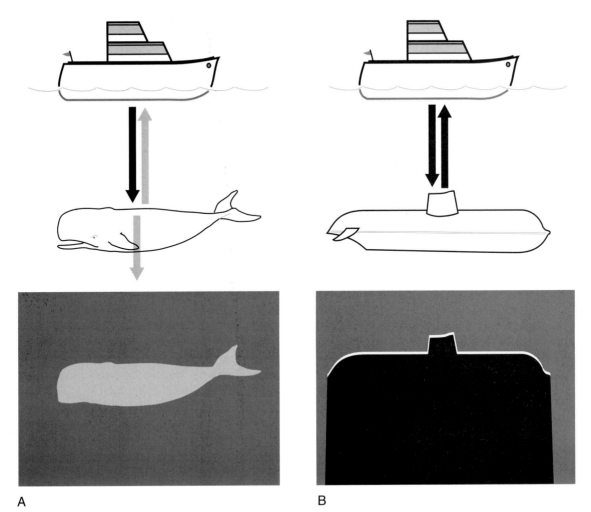

Figure 1–10. *A* and *B*, Various densities. A comparison of the ultrasound appearances of objects of the same size but of different densities. The metal submarine in *B* is more highly reflective than the whale in *A*.

vice capable of taking many frames per second, the sonar technician could soon learn to distinguish one type of whale from another and perhaps even individual whales from one another. The characteristic echoes formed by different types of schools of fish could be noted and important observations on the behavior of sea life could be recorded. Figure 1–11 gives some indication of what signals might be obtained.

Diagnostic ultrasound for medical purposes has followed a somewhat analogous course. The evolution from crude, one-dimensional images to composite images formed by multiple, serial scans to true, two-dimensional images able to detect motion in real time progressed rapidly over the past three decades. Before examining the images, however, we must consider the characteristics and terminology relating to the scanning devices themselves.

BASIC INSTRUMENTATION

Transducer Arrays

Ultrasound devices all use the same basic principle for generating the ultrasound waves and for receiving the reflected echoes. This is made possible by a property that quartz (and some other compounds) possesses, called the *piezoelectric effect*. There are actually two parts to this effect, both of which are critical for the function of diagnostic ultrasound. First, when the piezoelectric substance is compressed (*piezo* comes from the Greek word meaning "pressed"), as by

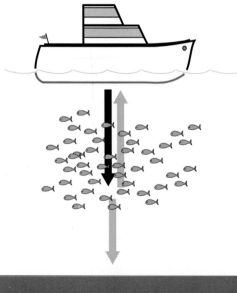

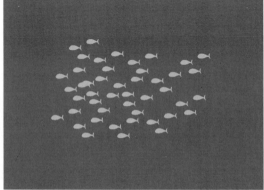

Figure 1–11. Different sizes. A group of fish swimming in the murky water below the boat produces a group of characteristic echoes that are distinctly different from the whale in Figure 1–10A, despite the similarity in tissue density between the fish and the whale.

a returning ultrasound wave, an electric current is generated. Conversely, when alternating electric current is applied to the piezoelectric element, the substance vibrates at a very stable frequency, and that frequency is a property of the substance used and its thickness. This duality of function allows for both transmission and reception of the ultrasound wave in one small instrument, referred to as the *transducer* or *probe*.

Many different arrangements of this basic piezoelectric transducer have been developed. Perhaps the simplest type conceptually is the *mechanical sector scanner*, which uses a single element that oscillates back and forth within the transducer head, as shown in Figure 1–12A. Some mechanical scanners use several transducers mounted on a wheel-like arrangement that rotates at a fixed speed within the head of the probe. This is illustrated schematically in Figure 1–12B; some examples of commercial transducers are shown in Figure 1–13. The basic mechanical scanners are relatively inexpensive and still used. Their focal length, however, is not variable (i.e., the ultrasound waves are focused at a fixed distance from the transducer head) and their vibration is noticeable to the operator and to the patient as well. A second type of transducer is referred to as a *linear array* or *sequential array* or *linear electronic scanner*. In this type of transducer, there is a sequential array of piezoelectric elements. As a result, the transducer head is generally longer than that of the mechanical sector scanner. The transducer

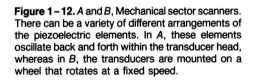

Figure 1–12. A and B, Mechanical sector scanners. There can be a variety of different arrangements of the piezoelectric elements. In A, these elements oscillate back and forth within the transducer head, whereas in B, the transducers are mounted on a wheel that rotates at a fixed speed.

A   B

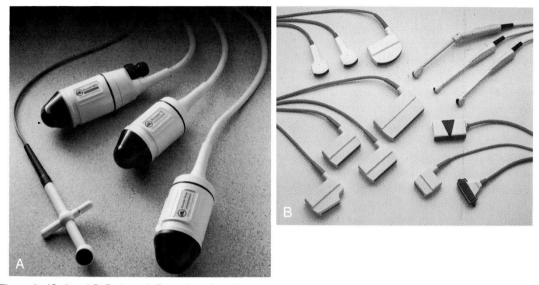

Figure 1–13. *A* and *B*, Probes. *A*, Examples of mechanical sector scanners and *B*, a variety of electronic transducers. (*A*, Courtesy of Advanced Technology Laboratories, Bothell, Washington; *B*, Courtesy of GE Medical Systems, Milwaukee, Wisconsin.)

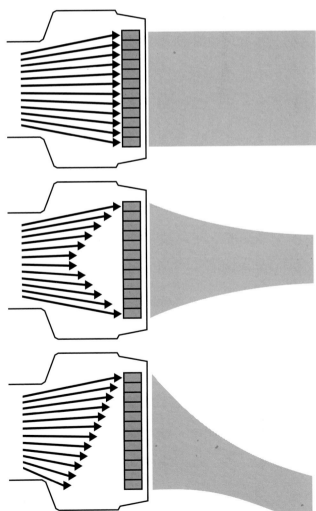

Figure 1–14. Linear array transducers. A large number of crystals are fired electronically in order to produce a sound beam from the probe. The focal length and direction of the beam can be changed by small differences in the sequence in which the crystals are fired.

head often contains more than 100 crystals, and these are fired electronically in groups to produce an ultrasound beam. The focal length and direction of this beam can be changed by varying the sequence in which the different crystals are activated; an example is illustrated schematically in Figure 1–14. Modern linear array scanners fire the entire sequence in a small fraction of a second, thereby allowing for real-time scanning in a manner similar to the mechanical sector scanners. The linear array scanner, as shown in Figure 1–15, produces an image that is rectangular, rather than the pie-shaped image produced by the mechanical sector scanner (Fig. 1–16). Compared to sector scanners, the electronic linear array scanners are more expensive and, for some applications, the long, narrow shape of the transducer head is a disadvantage. The *electronic sector scanner*, as illustrated in Figure 1–17, combines the advantages of the electronic circuitry of the linear electronic scanner, but the arrangement of the piezoelectric elements allows for a smaller transducer head. The main disadvantage is the greater cost. Yet another arrangement of transducers is referred to as an *annular array*. In this arrangement, the piezoelectric elements are arranged in a circular fashion around a central bull's eye. These are modestly priced and offer electronic focusing and a sector-shaped image. A final type of mod-

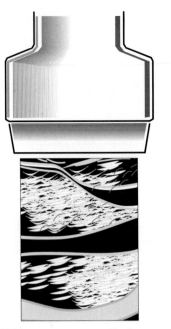

Figure 1–15. Linear array scanner. Produces a rectangular-shaped image.

ern transducer is known as the *curved linear scanner*. As shown in Figure 1–18, this transducer has a convex head that is smaller than the linear electronic scanner head, but the transducer is otherwise similar. It is capable of pro-

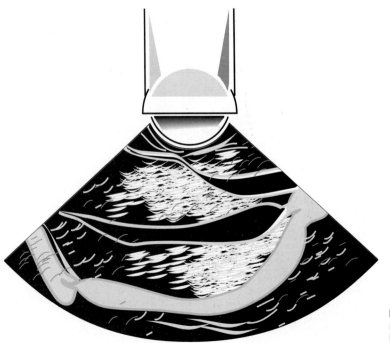

Figure 1–16. Mechanical sector scanner. Produces a pie-shaped image.

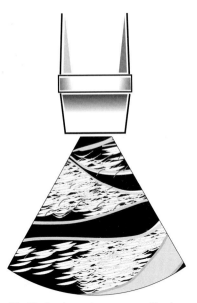

Figure 1–17. Electronic sector scanner. Produces a pie-shaped image.

in active use. One type of scanner that is virtually obsolete and is not suited for emergency medicine use is the *contact* or *static scanner*. This is quite a different instrument from the others and was once extensively used in obstetric and abdominal scanning; many images from this type of scanner are still found in textbooks and may be confusing, because they look quite different from those generated by more modern devices. This type of scanner has a long, moveable arm that is used to position the probe at a predetermined angle on the patient's skin. In the course of a relatively long time (several seconds at least), the static image is developed electronically from several images taken at different angles. Complexity, cost, and lack of real-time capability are serious disadvantages; the very large visual field obtained can be quite striking, and images from this device can be useful in demonstrating and teaching ultrasound anatomy.

Other Transducer Characteristics

In addition to the differences in the arrangement of the piezoelectric elements within the transducer head, there are other differences among transducers that are more relevant and more easily understood by the clinician. Trans-

viding excellent images, particularly in the near field, due to the convex shape of the head. The main disadvantages are that it may be awkward while scanning over a convex region and may be more expensive than some simpler arrangements.

All the transducers noted above are currently

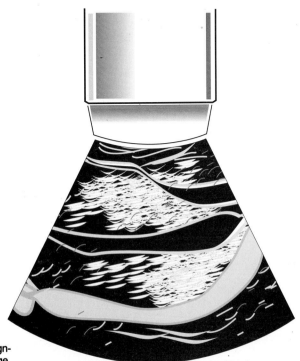

Figure 1–18. Curved linear array scanner. A convex alignment of transducer crystals produces the displayed image.

ducer frequency is a fairly straightforward concept that must be understood by any clinician who uses ultrasound. As noted earlier, ultrasound frequencies of use in medical imaging are in the megahertz (million hertz) range. For most clinical purposes, including emergency medicine use, transducer frequencies range from 3.0 to 7.5 MHz; specialized, non–emergency department applications, including ophthalmologic and intravascular ultrasound, use even higher frequency transducers.

The general principle is simple: other things being equal, *the higher the frequency, the greater the resolution and the less the penetration.* Therefore, for scanning of rather deep structures in adults, 3.5 MHz is often most appropriate. In many patients, the aorta and pelvic structures can be visualized best with a transducer of this frequency. Conversely, in thin patients and in children, visualization of abdominal and pelvic structures is often possible with a 5-MHz transducer, which allows for greater resolution and therefore better visualization of the anatomy. High-resolution transducers, usually defined as 7.5 MHz and greater, have some specific uses in emergency medicine, because small, superficial structures can be visualized. As discussed in Chapter 3 of this book, such probes are ideal for identification and removal of superficial foreign bodies, for testicular scanning, as an aid to suprapubic aspiration in infants, and for guided vascular applications. Commonly used transducer frequencies for various emergency conditions are summarized in Table 1–1. These are discussed in further detail throughout the text.

Table 1–1. COMMONLY USED TRANSDUCER FREQUENCIES

Transducer Frequency (MHz)		
3–3.5	5	7.5
Renal	Pediatric	Vascular
Aorta	abdominal exam	Foreign body
Gallbladder	Transvaginal exam	Transvaginal exam
Abdominal	Pediatric	Testicular
trauma	abdominal	
Cardiac	trauma	
Transabdominal	Testicular	
gynecologic		
exam		

Summary of Instrumentation

Figures 1–19 and 1–20 summarize the electronic steps involved in producing a real-time ultrasound image. The issues related to equipment selection for emergency department scanning are dealt with more fully in Appendix 1. The frequency of probes is only one of many factors that determine image quality and resolution. The arrangement of the piezoelectric crystals, the shape of the transducer footplate, and the characteristics of the focal length all affect transducer function significantly. Differences in the hardware and software of the scanner itself (discussed below) vary even more.

UNDERSTANDING THE FORMED IMAGE

Several conventions have been almost universally adopted for translating the electrical information generated by the transducer's piezoelectric effect to a two-dimensional image on the scanner screen.

The image is displayed so that the area nearest the transducer is at the top of the screen. This is true regardless of the shape of the image depicted. This convention is not necessarily used for certain specialized techniques, such as transvaginal, prostatic, and endovascular scan-

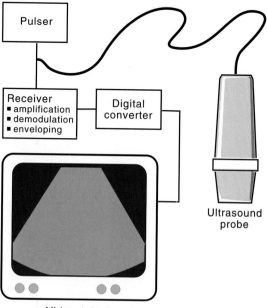

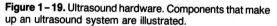

Figure 1–19. Ultrasound hardware. Components that make up an ultrasound system are illustrated.

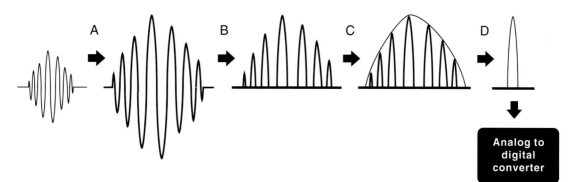

Figure 1-20. Electronic processing. There are a variety of electronic steps that the returning echo undergoes prior to being displayed on the ultrasound screen. *A*, Amplification; *B*, demodulation; *C*, enveloping; *D*, processing.

ning. Figures 1–15 to 1–18 show images from a rectangular linear array scanner, sector scanner, phased array scanner, and curved linear array scanner, respectively.

By convention, the *transverse scan* is presented so that the *patient's right-hand side is on the left side of the screen*. In other words, the cross-sectional view is depicted as though the slice were viewed standing at the patient's feet and looking cephalad, as depicted in Figure 1–21. This commonsense convention ensures that, if one had a large enough scanner, the left

side of the screen would demonstrate the right lobe of the liver progressing more medially to the kidney and, in order, the inferior vena cava, aorta, and then, to the far right-hand side of the screen, the left kidney. For *sagittal* use, the orientation is such that the patient's *cephalad part is on the left side of the screen* (Fig. 1–22). In a hypothetical case, this would mean that in an immense longitudinal scan of the abdomen at the left mid-clavicular line, the liver would be seen at the extreme left, followed by the gallbladder, appendix, and right ovary. In the mid-line, the

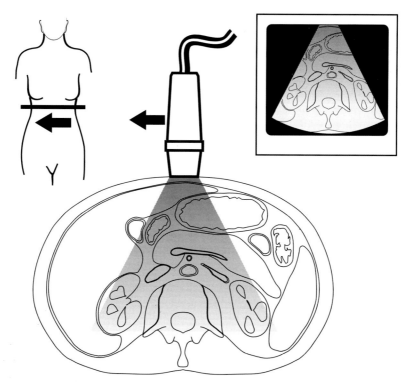

Figure 1-21. Standard transverse scan. This is obtained by directing the marker dot toward the patient's right-hand side. The patient's right side is depicted on the left side of the screen, as if viewed standing at the patient's feet.

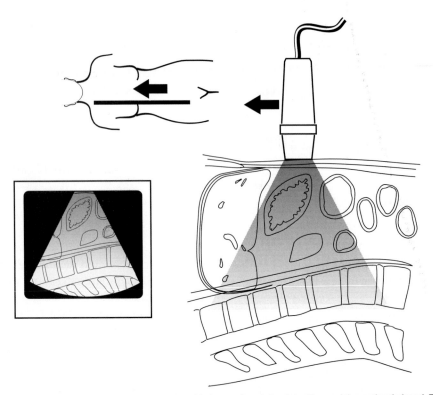

Figure 1–22. Standard longitudinal scan. The view with the marker dot pointed toward the patient's head. The cephalad portion of the patient is depicted on the left side of the screen (wherever the marker dot is pointing is on the left side of the screen).

aorta would seem to taper from the left-hand side of the screen as it goes distally toward the right-hand side of the screen.

To obtain this conventional view, it is necessary to know the orientation of the transducer's beam. All probes have incorporated a visual and/or palpable indicator, usually an indentation or an elevation that can easily be felt by the examiner's finger. *When scanning in the cross-sectional plane, this marker must point to the patient's right side.* In other words, if the examiner is positioned (as most North American physicians are accustomed) on the side of the patient's right arm, the marker groove is pointed toward the examining physician. When scanning in the longitudinal plane (i.e., a sagittal section), the marker groove must point to the patient's head. Another way of saying this is that *the marker groove always points to the left side of the screen* (for standard abdominal and pelvic scanning in North America), as demonstrated in Figures 1–21 and 1–22.

Gray Scale Versus White

In the earliest kind of sonogram, such as that generated by the device in Figure 1–23, the presence or absence of an object was predominantly an all-or-nothing affair. An echo is depicted at an appropriate distance on a one-dimensional graph (a line) that represents the sonographic beam. When multiple one-dimensional images are taken sequentially and the dots are connected, the tracing produced can be used to represent the contours of the ocean floor or the presence or absence of an enemy submarine. When a similar technique is used for medical imaging (now almost exclusively used for echocardiography), it is referred to as M-mode and the reflections are depicted as an "ice pick" view of the heart. Figure 1–24 illustrates an M-mode echocardiogram; as most physicians are aware, this type of study can be used to measure chamber size and valve motion and to document fetal viability and the like. With the added

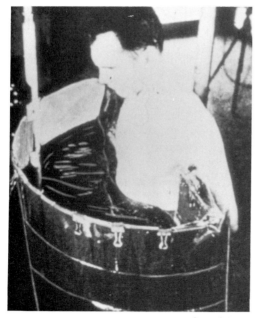

Figure 1–23. Early ultrasound equipment. One of the earliest ultrasound machines, which utilized a water bath in order to obtain ultrasound images. (Courtesy of Susan Beaulieu.)

complexity of true two-dimensional images, the ability to distinguish not just total absorption or total reflection of the ultrasound wave, but differences in the amount of ultrasonic reflection and absorption, results in an image that is far different. Like the sonar technician (see earlier

discussion) who learned to distinguish whales from submarines based on the character of the reflected sonar beam, the medical imager will find it necessary to display *gray scale* images in a conventional and consistent manner so that recognition of typical patterns can be achieved more regularly and so that images from different devices and different sonographers can be compared.

An object that reflects virtually *all* the ultrasound waves back toward the transducer (some gallstones, for example) is depicted as *white*. Because it is generating many echoes, it is referred to as *hyperechoic* (or sonodense). The opposite extreme, an object that transmits all the ultrasound impulses through it (a fluid-filled bladder, for example), has no reflectivity and is therefore referred to as *anechoic* (or sonolucent): it is depicted as pure *black*. These two extremes are illustrated in Figures 1–2 and 1–3. Gas-filled objects neither transmit nor reflect ultrasound waves in a useful manner and have no clear characterizations. The vast majority of structures have some degree of echogenicity and this, together with its internal architecture, forms patterns that are readily recognized with some experience. These can be quantitated mathematically but for clinical purposes are spoken of in a relative way such as "the liver looks more hyperechoic (or hypoechoic) than is usual" or "there is a 2-cm region of decreased

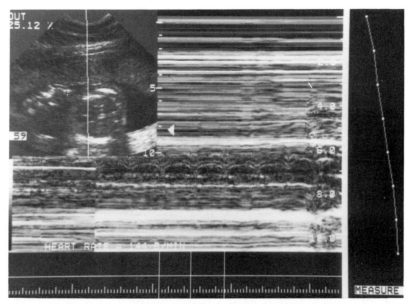

Figure 1–24. M-mode scan. This image documents fetal viability and heart rate. Motion is documented on the vertical axis and time on the horizontal axis.

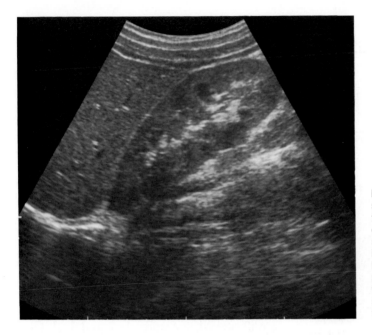

Figure 1–25. Normal kidney. The ultrasound appearance of the right kidney in the longitudinal (sagittal) plane. The renal capsule appears as an echogenic line surrounding the kidney. The renal cortex is slightly less echogenic than the neighboring liver, and the renal pyramids appear as hypoechoic areas that point toward the center of the kidney. The renal sinus is the central echogenic portion of the kidney.

echogenicity in an otherwise normal-appearing parenchyma.''

It is not always intuitively obvious why some structures appear as they do on ultrasound. Figure 1–25, for example, illustrates a normal kidney. A hyperechoic jagged white stripe is easily visible and is recognized as the intrarenal collecting system. This structure appears to be more echoic than the surrounding parenchyma because the connective tissue and peripelvic fat that comprise the collecting system are relatively more dense and have more reflective surfaces than does that of the surrounding parenchyma. Similarly, the diaphragm (Figure 1–26) routinely appears as a hyperechoic structure, particularly as compared to the adjacent liver. In

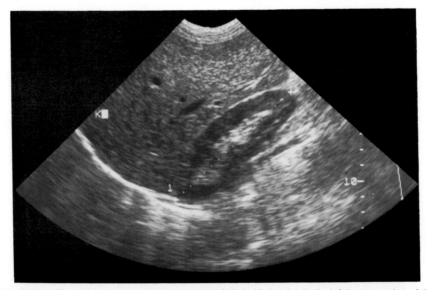

Figure 1–26. Diaphragm. The diaphragm appears as a hyperechoic (white) stripe in the left lower portion of the image. It is below and immediately adjacent to the liver. The hepatic veins appear as thin-walled structures that tend to run vertically (exception: right hepatic vein is more horizontal) in the liver (left of center of image), whereas the bile ducts and portal veins have echogenic walls and a more horizontal course (right upper portion of image). The markers to the right measure the length of the kidney.

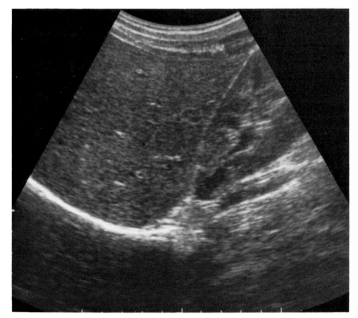

Figure 1–27. Normal liver. The liver has a relatively homogeneous appearance in this longitudinal scan. It is slightly more echogenic than the neighboring renal cortex.

this case the composition of the diaphragm owes its appearance to the presence of fatty tissue with many more reflective surfaces than the liver parenchyma. Figures 1–27 and 1–28 show two views of two different livers: the one with fatty infiltration (Fig. 1–28) has a slight increase in echoes relative to the normal liver (Fig. 1–27).

Gain

Gain refers to the amplification of the received signal and is an important concept in ultrasound imaging. Particularly when dealing with relative degrees of echogenicity, it is important to understand how gain affects the image. The electric impulse produced by the piezoelectric effect is ordinarily weak; in order to form an

Figure 1–28. Fatty infiltration of the liver. The liver demonstrates increased echogenicity. This is usually apparent in patients with moderate to severe fatty infiltration. As this process progresses, there is impaired visualization of the intrahepatic vessels, and the renal cortex appears relatively hypoechoic in comparison to the liver. The fatty infiltration may be nonuniform in its distribution within the liver. Causes of fatty infiltration include alcoholism, diabetes mellitus, obesity, steroid therapy, hyperlipidemia, hepatitis, parenteral nutrition, protein malnutrition, and ulcerative colitis.

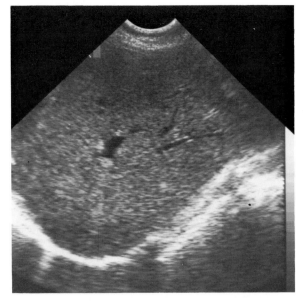

image on the ultrasound monitor, it must be boosted many times. This artificial increase in signal strength is referred to as gain, and it can markedly affect the appearance, particularly the perceived echogenicity, of almost all structures. Because gain is in fact the amount of amplification added to the signal coming from the transducer to the screen, *all parts of the image on the screen will be equally affected*. For nonradiologists, this would be somewhat comparable to the degree of penetration on a standard x-ray. Just as it is at times difficult to be sure if a chest radiograph is overpenetrated or whether the lucent appearance of the lung field is due to some degree of hyperaeration, judgments regarding gain also have a subjective element. Ordinarily, one can approximate the correct degree of echogenicity by comparing the reflectivity of certain structures of known sonodensity. There are times, however, where a degree of abnormal echogenicity might be attributable to a generalized physiologic condition (e.g., edematous states), rather than to too much amplification of the basic signal. Figure 1–29 illustrates three similar views of a normal liver with different degrees of gain. In this instance, Figure 1–29A with proper gain settings looks less sonodense than Figure 1–29B, where the gain was deliberately set too high, and more sonodense than Figure 1–29C, where the gain is set too low. However, viewing the liver alone, without other organs for comparison, it would be difficult to state that unequivocally. Figure 1–30 demonstrates a different liver with increased echogenicity from a patient with cirrhosis in which the gain was carefully set. The potential for misdiagnosis should be clear, because inappropriate gain settings can result in confusing images.

One of the direct consequences of the fact that ultrasound technology uses reflected rather than transmitted signals is that signals reflected from deeper in the tissue (which appear as being in the far field, or bottom of the screen) are much more attenuated by their passage through tissue than those situated more superficially. Although modern ultrasound devices compensate for this in their internal circuitry, the amount of attenuation is not constant (it depends on tissue characteristics), and manual fine tuning to obviate this discrepancy is often required. The *time gain compensator* (TGC) is present in some form on virtually all ultrasound devices. Unlike the gain control, it allows for selective enhancement or diminution of the reflectivity of a part of the image. The TGC is used when it is perceived that the gain in one part of the image compared to another part of the image is unequal. Ordinarily, the TGC is adjusted so that all parts of a reasonably large and homogeneous organ have equal gain, as illustrated in Figure 1–31. Again, there are pitfalls in this process; the perceived abnormality in reflectivity might in fact represent a true increase or decrease in echogenicity due to a pathologic process.

Axial and Lateral Resolution

Figures 1–32 and 1–33 demonstrate the difference between axial and lateral resolution of an object using ultrasound. The influence of beam width, frequency, pulse duration, and damping on resolution is illustrated in Figures 1–34 to 1–37.

EFFECTS AND ARTIFACTS

Both the basic laws of physics and particulars of the technology that is used to form, receive, and depict ultrasound waves lead to the production of images on the screen that can mislead or even startle the examiner. These phenomena may be true image artifacts (i.e., images occurring in a position or with some characteristic that does reflect the true anatomic state); at other times, there is no true artifact but the image obtained differs sufficiently from what is anticipated that there is difficulty in interpreting the ultrasound image. Because both effects and true artifacts can seriously diminish the usefulness of the ultrasound examination, the clinical distinction is perhaps not of great importance. Their recognition, however, is. The technical cause of some of these phenomena are remarkably complex, and the emphasis here is on recognition of how the particular effect appears on ultrasound images and identification of those times in emergency practice when they are likely to occur.

Central Image Effects
Acoustic Shadowing

Acoustic shadowing is one of the easiest of all characteristic ultrasound effects to understand and is of particular importance in several common emergency examinations, both as an aid to

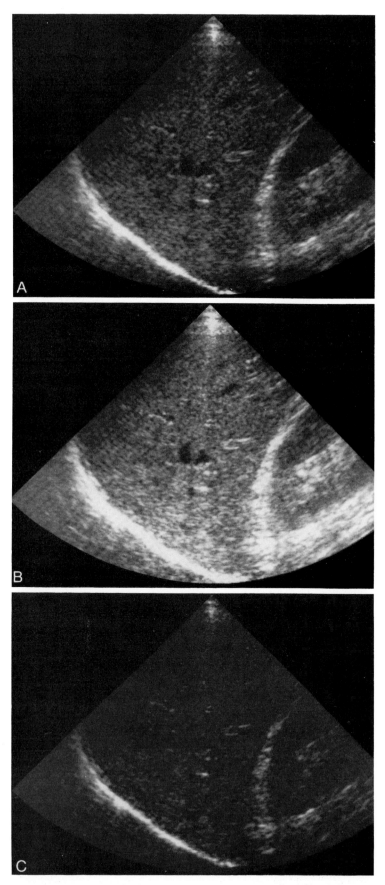

Figure 1–29. *A–C,* Normal liver with different gain settings. *A,* Proper gain settings. All the gray scale bars to the far left of the screen will be visible. *B,* Excessive brightness; the gray scale bars will no longer be visible. *C,* The gain is set too low, which will result in a suboptimal gray bar display. (From Sanders RC: Clinical Sonography: A Practical Guide, 2nd ed. Boston: Little, Brown, 1991:484.)

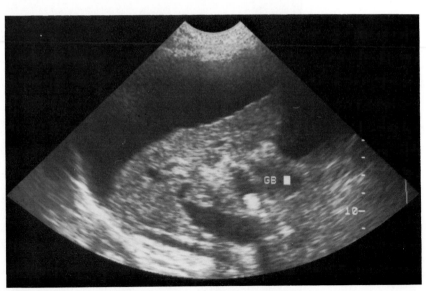

Figure 1–30. Cirrhosis. There is increased echogenicity of the liver parenchyma. The cirrhotic liver is usually small, with an irregular border and surrounded by ascitic fluid (dark).

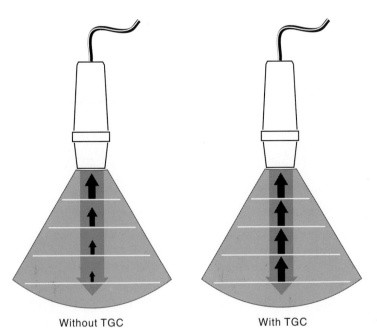

Without TGC   With TGC

Figure 1–31. Time-gain compensation (TGC). This is normally set so that all parts of a homogeneous organ will have equivalent brightness. The time-gain compensation is used to compensate for the loss of amplitude that occurs due to attenuation of the sound wave as it passes through the tissue. Most ultra-sound devices allow the sonographer to adjust the degree of time-gain compensation to correspond to the degree of attenuation in the tissue.

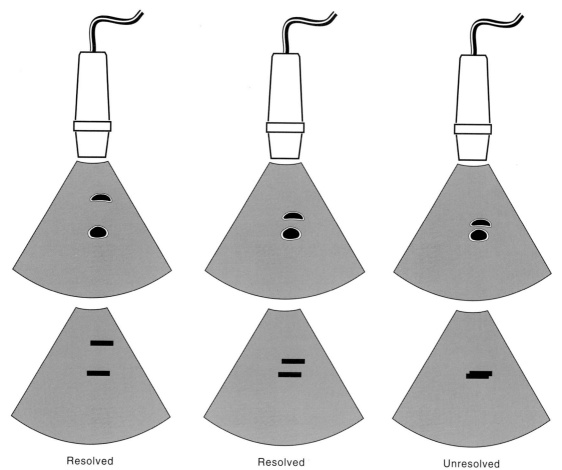

Resolved   Resolved   Unresolved

Figure 1–32. Axial resolution. The ability to distinguish closely spaced objects along the axis of the ultrasound beam.

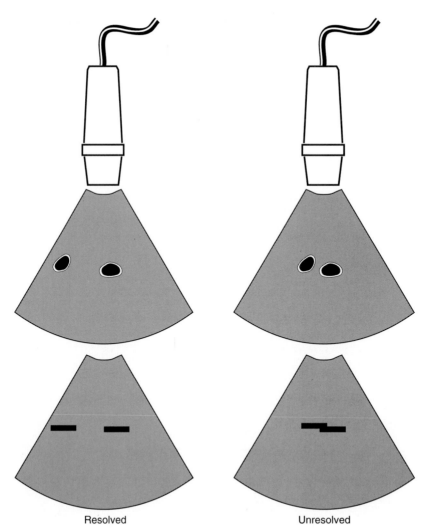

Resolved   Unresolved

Figure 1 – 33. Lateral resolution. The ability to distinguish closely spaced objects along an axis perpendicular to that of the ultrasound beam.

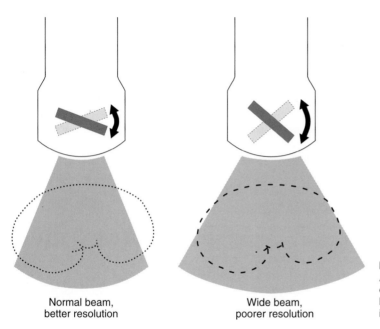

Normal beam,
better resolution

Wide beam,
poorer resolution

Figure 1 – 34. Beam width on resolution. As the angle of the sector scanner is decreased, the field of view becomes more limited; however, the resolution of the image improves.

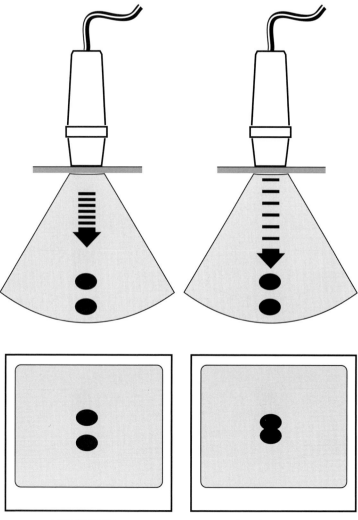

High frequency   Low frequency

Figure 1–35. Transducer frequency on axial resolution. When operating at a lower frequency with the same number of cycles, the spatial pulse length is increased, thereby diminishing the axial resolution.

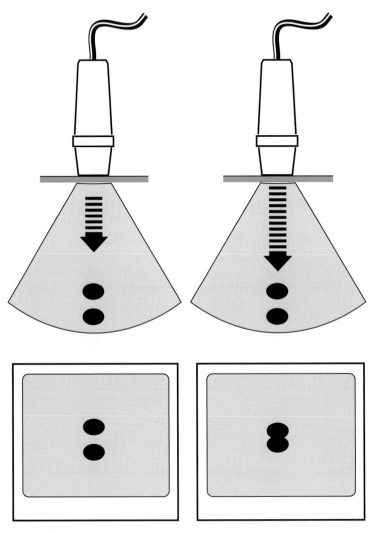

Short pulse duration   Long pulse duration

Figure 1–36. Pulse duration on axial resolution. A larger number of cycles of the same frequency produce a longer pulse duration, which decreases the axial resolution.

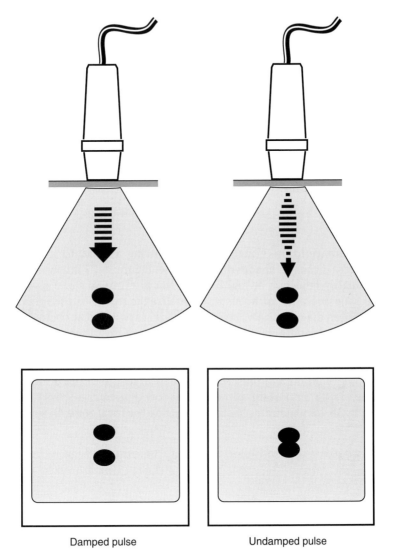

Damped pulse   Undamped pulse

Figure 1–37. Pulse dampening on axial resolution. Dampening decreases the pulse length, thereby improving the axial resolution.

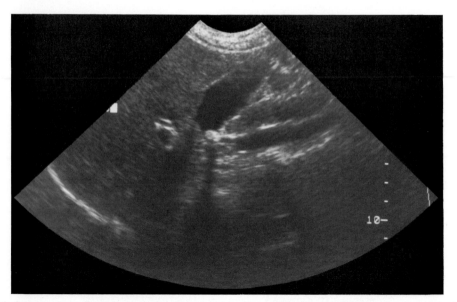

Figure 1–38. Gallstone. An echogenic structure seen in the neck of the gallbladder with posterior acoustic shadowing, which represents a gallstone.

diagnosis and as a hindrance to the visualization of distal structures. Acoustic shadowing occurs distal to any highly reflective or highly attenuating surface. The presence of acoustic shadowing is an important diagnostic clue seen in a large number of medical conditions, including biliary stones, renal stones, and tissue calcifications. Recognition of the acoustic shadow, which may be much more prominent than the underlying substrate, is an important ultrasound clue. Figure 1–38 demonstrates distal

shadowing related to a well-visualized gallstone. Figure 1–39 illustrates a similar case, but in this instance no stone is visible. Failure to visualize the source of a shadow can be caused by several factors. Most commonly, it is related to the plane of the ultrasound beam in comparison to that of the small, reflective object. As shown in Figures 1–40 and 1–41, an object at or near the focal length of the ultrasound beam casts a shadow of greater intensity than if the object is outside the focal zone. In such a situation, care-

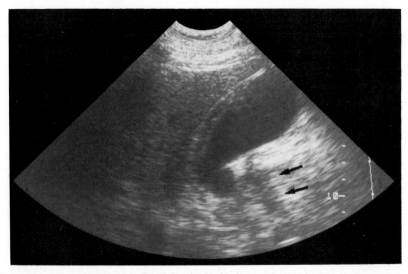

Figure 1–39. Shadowing without visible stone. Posterior shadowing is seen (*arrows*) without evidence of a stone within the gallbladder.

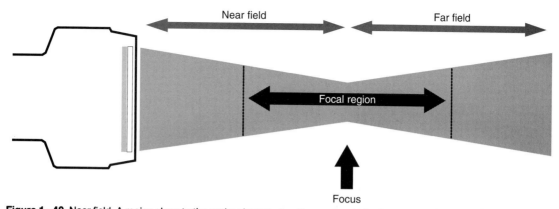

Figure 1–40. Near field. A region close to the probe characterized by great variation in ultrasound intensity from one wave to the next. The far field, in contrast, has more uniform intensity between wavefronts; however, the wavefronts start to diverge. The best imaging is obtained in the area where we see a transition between the near field and the far field (focal region).

ful scanning through planes only slightly different from that initially used ordinarily reveals the object. Figure 1–42 demonstrates this effect in the same patient as in Figure 1–39. By scanning at only a minimally different angle, both the shadow and the stone are readily visible. At times, the condition of the surrounding tissue may make visualization of the object difficult or impossible. Small stones within the echogenic but shrunken or scarred gallbladder (Fig. 1–43A) or bile-containing ducts (Fig. 1–43B) may be difficult or impossible to differentiate from the surrounding tissue.

Acoustic shadowing may also cause confusion by its absence when it might otherwise be expected. Figure 1–44 demonstrates what seems to be several small gallstones (next to gallstones that shadow), but no shadowing is demonstrated. This is likely to occur in situations where the reflective object is small or located far from the focal point of the ultrasound beam. The shadow can be maximized by using a transducer of higher frequency and by adjusting the focal point.

A final, more subtle problem with acoustic shadowing is worth mentioning. Total acoustic shadowing by a completely reflective object may obscure distal structures, but the operator will be aware of the problem due to the easily visible margins of the shadow. If the region is

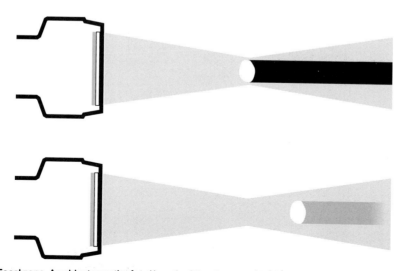

Figure 1–41. Focal zone. An object near the focal length of the ultrasound beam casts a much more distinct or cleaner shadow than that cast by the same object when it is located outside of the focal zone.

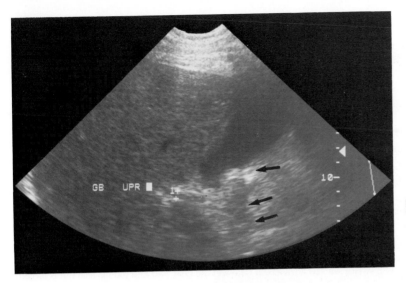

Figure 1 – 42. Gallstone shadowing. The same patient as in Figure 1 – 39 is scanned at a slightly different angle; both the ''dirty'' shadow (*lower arrows*) and stone (*upper arrow*) are now visible.

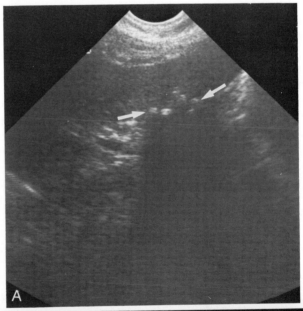

Figure 1 – 43. *A*, Stones in a contracted gallbladder. Small stones (*arrows*) in a shrunken gallbladder can be very difficult to differentiate from surrounding tissue. There is prominent acoustic shadowing distal to these stones. *B*, Stones in common bile duct. Two echogenic gallstones with posterior shadowing are visualized in a dilated common bile duct.

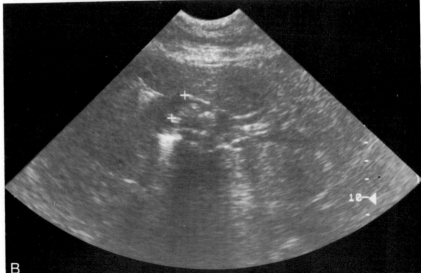

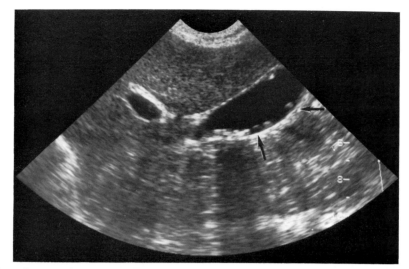

Figure 1–44. Posterior acoustic shadowing. There are several gallstones that shadow poorly in the gallbladder (*arrows*). In addition, there are multiple gallstones in the left portion of the gallbladder adjacent to the neck that demonstrate good posterior acoustic shadowing.

only somewhat more reflective than the surrounding tissue, *partial shadowing* occurs, which may not be so obvious. Although not a major problem in the usual focused emergency department examination, it is not difficult to see how regions of mild attenuation (decreased echoes) distal to a relatively hyperechoic lesion could be overlooked. The interface between tissue and air acts much like a highly reflective object in terms of producing acoustic shadowing. A most common example of this—and the bane of abdominal scanning—is caused by

gas-filled loops of bowel. Such shadows may be large and difficult or impossible to get around, but they are ordinarily obvious to the scanner. Shadows from small bubbles of gas within the bowel are less striking, but can scatter the ultrasound waves and seriously degrade the image. Figure 1–45 illustrates the shadow from the splenic flexure partly obscuring the kidney: this is a routine occurrence. Occasionally, identification of an acoustic shadow caused by gas in the wall of an organ that does not normally contain gas will lead to an important diagnosis.

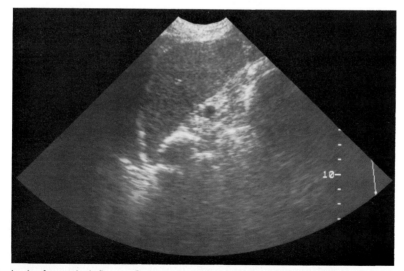

Figure 1–45. Shadowing from splenic flexure. Gas present in the splenic flexure results in "dirty" acoustic shadowing, seen in the right upper portion of this image. This is a common occurrence that may interfere with visualization of the left kidney. Moving the probe to a slightly more posterior location usually allows full visualization of the left kidney.

Figure 1–46 illustrates this phenomenon in a case of emphysematous cholecystitis. Gas-produced shadowing of this type is often less distinct at the margins than that produced by calcium or large gallstones; therefore, this shadowing is sometimes referred to as "dirty shadows," as opposed to the sharp-edged shadows, which are said to be "clean."

Acoustic Enhancement

Acoustic enhancement is a very important phenomenon that can be observed to some degree in almost every scan. In fact, good scanning techniques for many emergency department indications deliberately make use of this effect. One way to think of acoustic enhancement is as the opposite of (partial) acoustic shadowing. Just as a relatively hyperechoic region to some extent blocks the transmission of ultrasound waves distal to it, an area of better ultrasound transmission allows enhancement of the ultrasound signal distal to that region. Figure 1–47A illustrates both acoustic shadowing and acoustic enhancement. The gallbladder is an anechoic structure analogous to a fluid-filled cyst. The

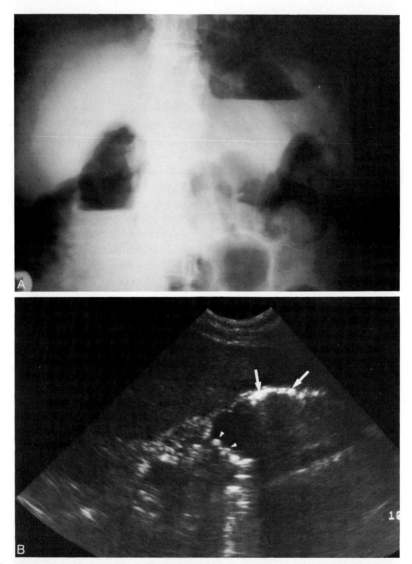

Figure 1–46. Emphysematous cholecystitis. *A*, The radiograph demonstrates an air–fluid level in the right upper quadrant consistent with the diagnosis of emphysematous cholecystitis. *B*, The ultrasound of the same patient demonstrates gallstones (*arrowheads*) in a dependent location with some posterior acoustic shadowing. The intraluminal gas (*arrows*) appears as a dense span of hyperechoic reflectors with some "comet-tail" shadowing.

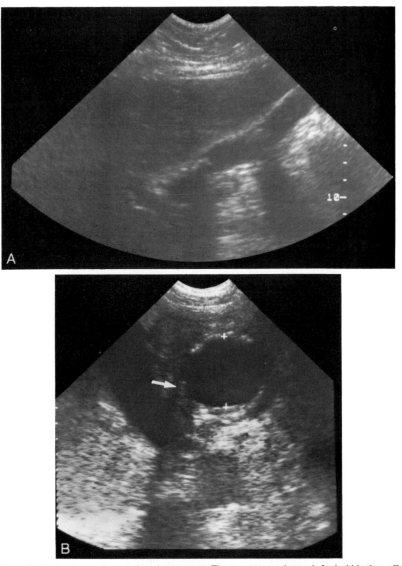

Figure 1–47. *A,* Acoustic shadowing and acoustic enhancement. There are two echogenic foci within the gallbladder that have posterior acoustic shadowing. The region distal to the fluid-filled portion of the gallbladder (without gallstones) demonstrates increased transmission of sound waves and appears brighter (with better resolution) than adjacent regions at similar depths. Cystic structures are frequently utilized as acoustic windows in order to make use of acoustic enhancement. *B,* Acoustic enhancement. This ultrasound image of a pancreatic pseudocyst demonstrates acoustic enhancement posterior to the fluid-filled cyst (between the two markers). In addition, there is acoustic enhancement distal to the gallbladder that appears in the left portion of the image. The wall of the pancreatic pseudocyst demonstrates lateral cystic shadowing (*arrow*), which produces a thin, dark shadow parallel to the direction of the ultrasound beam and tangential to the wall of the cyst.

region distal to this cyst-like structure has a relatively increased transmission of ultrasound waves and therefore appears lighter (more white) than adjoining regions. Visualization of the region distally to the fluid-filled structure is actually enhanced.

The term *acoustic window* is used somewhat generally to indicate a scanning position that is particularly favorable for visualizing the structure of interest. Many cystic structures can serve as acoustic windows. Figure 1–47*B* is one of a great many in this book that illustrates the appearance of acoustic enhancement on ultrasound images. A common beginner's mistake is to confuse this area of increased echogenicity for a true tissue lesion.

Lateral Cystic Shadowing

Yet another interesting effect occurs in relation to cystic structures and blood vessels. As shown in Figures 1–47B and 1–48, a thin shadow may extend from the lateral edges of the cystic structure being scanned. At least one of the several reasons for this phenomenon is that refraction of ultrasound waves occurs on absorption at the cyst's surface, leading to a region with relatively few ultrasound waves, especially compared to the enhanced transmission directly deep to the cystic structure. Figure 1–4 and the earlier discussion in the section Sound and Ultrasound may clarify this slightly arcane phenomenon. The important point is that such shadows may appear adjacent to the gallbladder, vessels, or ducts and can easily mimic the shadows caused by stones or intramural gas. Unlike calculi-induced shadows, however, these shadows are always parallel to the direction of the ultrasound beam and tangential to the wall of the cystic structure. Visualization in at least two planes should obviate the problem.

Artifacts

Hundreds of ultrasound artifacts have been described. Fortunately, the vast majority are either very rare or apply to specific areas of the anatomy. The artifacts discussed here are those that are either quite common or that have particular importance to standard emergency sonographic studies. It must be reemphasized that the causes of many of the effects and artifacts are often complex and variable. All explanations presented here are simplifications.

There are several ultrasound artifacts that are similar in the sense that they all result from the erroneous projection of some outlying structure within a second organ, thus simulating the appearance of disease. This can occur if two structures in the same ultrasound path take significantly different amounts of time to be reflected back to the transducer head. Because the image on the screen is artificially constructed with the assumption that there is a direct relationship between increasing time for echo return and increasing distance from the probe, the common element in all these artifacts is that distal and proximal structures are superimposed. The reasons for this time discrepancy vary and are often quite technical, but include such factors as interference between ultrasound waves, reflection of ultrasound waves, tissue interfaces, and the extremely close proximity of tissues with very different transmission characteristics.

Beam-Width Artifact

"Pseudo sludge" is an example of the common beam-width artifact. When the focal zone of the transducer is at the center of the gallbladder, the

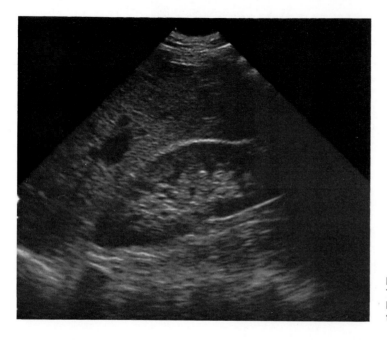

Figure 1–48. Lateral cystic shadowing. There is a fluid-filled structure (vein) in the liver that produces shadowing tangential to its wall.

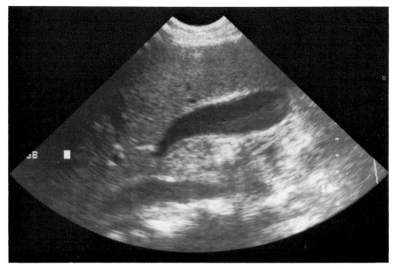

Figure 1–49. Pseudo sludge. This artifact results from a partial volume effect along the posterior wall of the gallbladder and produces an appearance similar to that of sludge.

beam is of greater width at the posterior border of the gallbladder. The partial volume effect along the posterior wall results in the appearance of particulate matter, or sludge, in the gallbladder. This phenomenon, which is easily visualized in real time, is illustrated in Figure 1–49.

Gas bubbles, which are very common in the duodenum, can be similarly projected adjacent to the gallbladder, simulating a gallstone. Figure 1–50 illustrates this phenomenon. The artifactual image differs from sludge and stones in that it does not assume a dependent posture and the lateral margins of the artifacts do not conform precisely to the walls of the gallbladder.

Side Lobe Artifacts

Figure 1–51 illustrates the fact that more than one beam is generated at the transducer head. Normally, these side lobes are of low intensity (1%) in comparison to the central axis of the beam and therefore are of little significance. Occasionally, these side lobes can cause artifacts, including the false projection of intestinal gas into the gallbladder, simulating disease. Figure 1–52 illustrates how the presence of a very reflective bowel–gas interface can return echoes to the transducer through side lobes, rather than through the normal path of the main ultrasound beam. This artifact may be obviated by alternating the angle of the transducer head, presumably preventing the echoes from reaching the weaker side lobes.

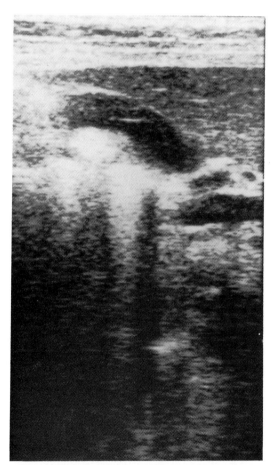

Figure 1–50. Gas simulating gallstones. There is a hyperechoic structure with weak posterior acoustic shadowing along the posterior wall of the gallbladder. This hyperechoic complex is actually a strong echo from intestinal gas adjacent to the gallbladder, not a gallstone. This artifact disappeared when scanned at different angles. (From Higashi Y, Mizushima A, Matsumoto H: Introduction to Abdominal Sonography. Berlin: Springer-Verlag, 1988:107.)

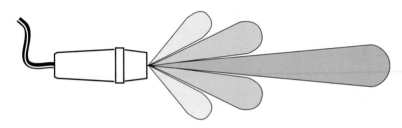

Figure 1-51. Side lobes. All ultrasound beams have side lobes, but these are generally of little consequence. The side lobes usually have intensities that are less than 1% of that of the central beam. The side lobes may occasionally result in some minor degradation of lateral resolution.

Reverberation Artifacts

There are several types of reverberation artifacts, all caused when the returning ultrasound beam bounces back and forth between two or more highly reflective surfaces. As a result, parallel bands of *reverberation echoes* are depicted on the image and are superimposed on whatever structure lies beneath the reflective layers;

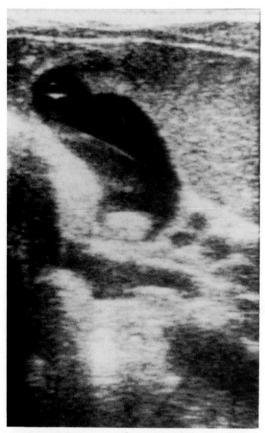

Figure 1-52. Side lobe artifact. Highly reflective bowel gas can return sound waves to the transducer through side lobes. This appears as an oblique line within the lumen of the gallbladder. These echoes disappear with minor changes in the angle of the transducer head. In addition, there is a gallstone noted in the dependent portion of the gallbladder. (From Higashi Y, Mizushima A, Matsumoto H: Introduction to Abdominal Sonography. Berlin: Springer-Verlag, 1988:21.)

the ultrasound device is fooled by the time delay (Fig. 1-53). Most commonly, the reflective layers are in the abdominal wall (Fig. 1-54A); however, many other reflectors, including gas (Fig. 1-46B) and foreign bodies (Fig. 1-54B) do the same. When the reverberations occur between two very closely spaced interfaces, multiple reverberations merge and a "comet-tail" pattern, illustrated in Figure 1-54B, is produced. Reverberation artifacts may be distracting, but are less likely to be confused with pathologic change than other artifacts.

The Mirror Effect

The striking *mirror effect* artifact occurs in the course of gallbladder or liver scanning when the ultrasound beam is reflected back into the liver by the diaphragm and bounces back again to the transducer head via the diaphragm. This results in the intrahepatic architecture being depicted as though it were cephalad to the diaphragm, as seen in Figures 1-55 and 1-56. This mirror image can be mistaken for thoracic disease.

Gain Artifacts

As mentioned previously, inappropriate settings of the gain or TGC (the control for adjusting gain in different parts of the field) have the potential to cause considerable confusion (Fig. 1-57). A problem common to beginners is the overuse of the gain or TGC to enhance contrast. When this is done, artifactual reflections can be produced in what should be an anechoic structure such as an ovarian cyst or urinary bladder, or, conversely, the distinctive tissue character of recognizable structures can be eliminated.

Contact Artifacts

Perhaps the least exciting and most common of all artifacts is that which is created when the transducer head makes only intermittent contact with the skin surface. A fairly typical pat-

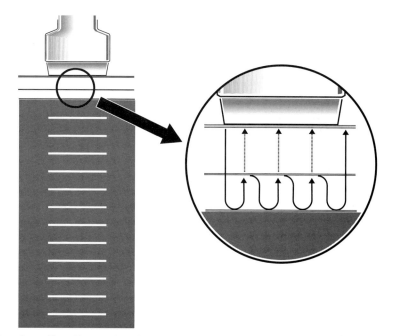

Figure 1–53. Reverberation artifact. Occurs when the ultrasound rays are bounced between two reflective layers. Causes of this artifact include metallic foreign bodies, cholesterol gallbladder stones, layers of the abdominal wall, and gas bubbles, to name a few.

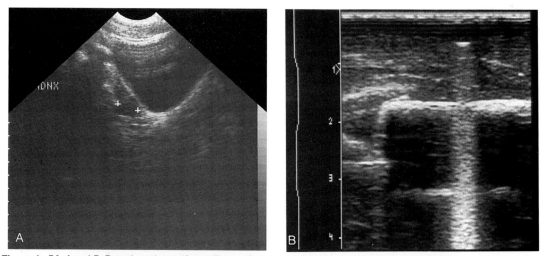

Figure 1–54. A and B, Reverberation artifacts. This artifact occurs as a result of ultrasound waves being bounced back and forth between two or more highly reflective surfaces. These reflective layers may be within the abdominal wall (A) or from a foreign body (B). If the reflective layers are very closely spaced, multiple reverberations merge and a "comet-tail" pattern (B) results.

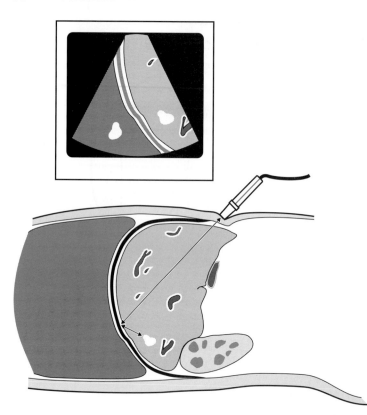

Figure 1–55. Mirror artifact. Occurs when the ultrasound beam undergoes multiple reflections prior to returning to the transducer. Occasionally, an image of an object may appear on both sides of the diaphragm due to this artifact (the deeper structure on the screen is the false image).

tern results when insufficient contact gel is used, as shown in Figure 1–58.

Artifacts and Effects: Summary

There is no substitute for experience in recognizing and minimizing ultrasound artifacts.

Table 1–2 summarizes common ultrasound artifacts encountered in emergency medicine practice, lists the common causes, and suggests solutions. Many other examples and much more rigorous treatments of the underlying physics are available in the standard texts cited in the Bibliography.

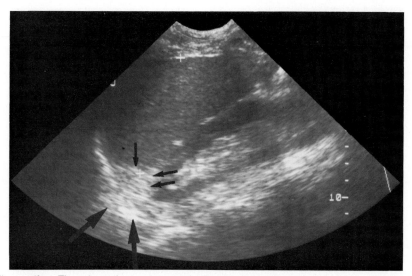

Figure 1–56. Mirror artifact. The echogenic structure proximal to the diaphragm (*small arrows*) is projected superior to the diaphragm (*large arrows*).

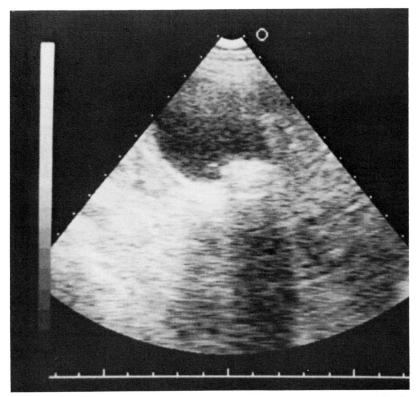

Figure 1–57. Gain artifact. The gain is set too high on this ultrasound image. The fluid in the gallbladder should have an anechoic appearance, but contains artifactual reflections as a result of the inappropriate gain settings. Shadowing from the gallstones has a ''dirty'' appearance as the result of the excessive gain settings.

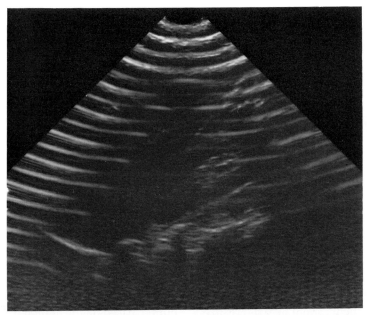

Figure 1–58. Contact artifact. This usually occurs as a result of applying inadequate amounts of ultrasound gel between the transducer and the skin surface.

Table 1-2. COMMON ULTRASOUND ARTIFACTS

Artifact	Cause	Solution
Pseudo sludge (beam-width artifact)	Echoes from adjacent organ (e.g., bowel) projected into nearby organ lumen (e.g., gallbladder)	Variation in patient position
Side lobe artifact	Echoes returning to transducer through side lobes rather than main beam	Alternating angle of transducer head; change type of transducer
Reverberation artifact (ring down artifact)	Reflection of beam between highly reflective surfaces results in parallel echoes of decreasing intensity	Variation of probe frequency and position
Mirror effect	Reflection of echoes from liver by diaphragm creates image above diaphragm	Visualization from different position; altering angulation of probe
Gain artifact	Inappropriate gain or time gain compensator (TGC) setting	Careful adjustment of gain using region of known echogenicity

SCANNING TECHNIQUES

Techniques relevant to the different scans pertinent to emergency medicine are covered in detail in Chapters 2 and 3. There are, however, some general techniques that are of universal applicability.

Patient Interaction

Ultrasound scanning, at least emergency ultrasound scanning, is not like taking a radiograph. The ultrasound probe is quite literally an extension of the clinician's hand, and the ultrasound examination is an extension of the history and physical examinations. The anatomic information provided by the ultrasound images is just one of the benefits, and not always the major benefit, of the interactive ultrasound study. The sonographic examination is brief, but it allows for an unparalleled opportunity to communicate with the patient in ways that are often not emphasized or overlooked entirely in the emergency department setting. Studies have indicated that patients' complaints regarding their care in emergency departments are not ordinarily related to their concern for the physician's competence, but rather center on the perception that the physician did not demonstrate his or her concern for the patient in the ways the patient expected: listening, talking, and examining. Emergency ultrasound is a powerful tool in part because the patient cannot help but realize that the physician is literally using his or her hands as well as technology in the patient's interest.

Most patients have some idea of what ultrasound is, but a few words at the outset to state that this is a safe and pain-free technique that will aid in the investigation of the problem is usually appropriate. In most cases, it is wise to position the screen so that the patient may view the examination if he or she desires (which is almost always the case). It is very common that, during the course of the ultrasound examination and ensuing discussion, a more focused history and physical examination will develop, allowing for a better definition of what kind of investigation is most appropriate. Pain and tenderness, which at first are thought to be localized to a classic region, often turn out to be quite different when investigated with the aid of ultrasound-guided palpation. Most often, the new area of interest can be investigated immediately, with the patient providing feedback. In many instances, the emergency department ultrasound examination, like the rest of the workup, may not give a definitive answer, but it is rare that ultrasound does not provide the clinician with more information. It is rarer still that the therapeutic milieu is not enhanced.

Move the Patient

The initial emergency department examination is almost always done with the patient in the supine position. Many times, this is all that is required, based on the limited nature of the emergency department studies performed. In cases where visualization is not optimal, however, significant questions may exist regarding an ultrasound appearance. Moving the patient from one position to another is often the single most important step in resolving the problem.

Rotate the Probe 90 Degrees

The simple act of obtaining images in two perpendicular planes should be routine for each area of interest. The nature of the structure in question (e.g., tubular versus cystic, aorta versus vena cava) is often resolved.

Apply Compression During Scanning

The application of firm but gentle pressure can remarkably improve the quality of ultrasound images. The distance to the target organ is often markedly decreased by compression, thereby allowing a more appropriate focal length or higher resolution transducer; intervening loops of bowel can sometimes be markedly compressed, and artifacts from bowel gas can be reduced or eliminated. Firm pressure may greatly improve the skin–transducer interface, particularly with rectangular-shaped transducers and when imaging over convex body parts.

Use the Patient's Respiration to Define Desired Structures

The remarkable degree of movement of the liver, spleen, kidney, and gallbladder is often unappreciated to those not performing ultrasound or fluoroscopy regularly. Holding the transducer steady in the transverse plane while the patient takes several deep breaths often results in rapid identification of the section of interest. In order to visualize intraperitoneal structures that lie below the rib cage, one can use the subcostal approach in conjunction with deep inspiration and protrusion of the anterior abdominal wall (the patient pushes his or her belly outward).

Change the Angle of the Transducer Prior to Repositioning

The ultrasound beam sweeps out in a fan-shaped fashion. Small changes in angulation result in large differences in the section being scanned.

Use Ultrasound During the Physical Examination

The use of transabdominal ultrasound during the standard manual examination can be edifying in terms of identification of fullness, masses, and areas of tenderness. The position of the examining finger ordinarily can be identified and structures thought previously to have been (for example) ovaries frequently prove to be something else. Ultrasound can be used in a similar way when examining masses or tenderness in the abdomen and scrotum.

Use the Highest Frequency Transducer That Will Visualize the Area of Interest

Many gallbladder, kidney, pelvic, and aorta examinations are significantly improved with a 5-MHz rather than 3.5-MHz transducer.

Obtain More Images on Hard Copy Than Are Absolutely Necessary

What appears on the hard copy is often an approximation, and a highly selected one at that, of information gained during the real-time examination. Often these extra views will settle an issue raised on review of the hard copy. In addition, views from emergency examinations are frequently reviewed and borrowed by the numerous consultants who may be asked to see the patient.

Use Compression Techniques, Valsalva Maneuver, and Posture

These maneuvers should be employed liberally when performing vascular scanning for either diagnosis or vascular access. These are also invaluable techniques during abdominal scanning in order to confirm the identity of large vessels and bowel.

Use a Spacer

An artificial acoustic window should be employed between the transducer and the skin surface if the structure being scanned is not at an optimal focal length. The spacer can be as simple as an examining glove filled with water or a prefabricated, commercial spacer. In either case, image quality is often greatly improved by providing this near-perfect acoustic window and repositioning the image in a favorable field.

Use the Intercostal Approach Freely

When the abdominal (especially gallbladder) scan is not optimal or when the patient is extremely tender, the intercostal approach is often the best option.

BIOLOGIC EFFECTS AND SAFETY CONSIDERATIONS

There is nothing inherent about the physics of ultrasound waves that make them immune from safety concerns. Although they use no ionizing radiation, it is clear that every ultrasound device transmits energy into the organism at which it is directed. The fact that this energy is capable of disrupting biologic systems may be inferred from the striking effects that high-energy ultrasound waves have when directed in a therapeutic fashion against renal or biliary stones. Because the major difference between these therapeutic units and diagnostic units are in their power (i.e., the rate at which energy is transmitted into the medium), it is reasonable to ask whether diagnostic medical ultrasound can pose any risk.

Several lines of investigation suggest that the biologic effects of ultrasound with current devices are so small as to be immeasurable. First, there is the epidemiologic evidence that no known ill effect has been thought to occur after several million ultrasound examinations. A more scientific approach is to examine the studies that have attempted to determine whether fetuses exposed to ultrasound in utero may have an increased incidence of some ill effect. These studies are difficult to do, not only because of the large numbers of patients that are needed, but also because of the difficulty in proving matched groups; patients subjected to ultrasound are often at greater risk due to underlying disease than those who are not scanned. Although such studies are ongoing, it is correct to say that there has been no evidence yet of a greater incidence of fetal abnormalities; evidence of genetic disruption (which might be manifested in the next generation) would clearly require many more years of study before being ruled out definitively. In studies on animals and particularly mammalian cells in vitro, no consistent result is clear. Almost all studies indicating any possibility of an effect on cell cultures have been obtained using time-averaged intensities or exposure times that bear no relation to the devices and times used in clinical sonography.

A fairly recent review by the American Institute of Ultrasound in Medicine (AIUM) concluded that, for focused ultrasound beams such as those used in medical diagnostic imaging, there was a very great margin of safety based on biologic effects related to energy output. A general policy has been enunciated and supported by governmental agencies that ultrasound examination should not be done in a frivolous manner, and use of "as low as reasonably attainable" exposure for a given study is a reasonable standard. There is no doubt that the use of diagnostic ultrasound for medical or research purposes is as safe as almost any clinical intervention imaginable. Certainly for the emergency physician in treating an acutely symptomatic patient, it would be difficult to imagine the situation where the theoretic and extraordinarily small risks of ultrasound would come close to outweighing the potential benefits of the study.

The official position of the AIUM is that "no confirmed biologic effects on patients or instrument operators caused by exposure at intensities typical of present diagnostic U/S instruments have ever been reported. Although the possibility exists that such biological effects may be identified in the future, current data indicates that the benefits of the prudent use of diagnostic ultrasound outweigh the risks, if any, that may be present."

BIBLIOGRAPHY

All the standard ultrasound texts have introductory chapters dealing with the fundamentals of ultrasound physics, instrumentation, artifacts, and bioeffects. All are far more detailed than the brief presentation in this chapter. Some are dauntingly mathematical.

Fleischer AC, James AE: Diagnostic Sonography: Principles and Clinical Applications. Philadelphia: W. B. Saunders, 1989.

Goldberg BB: Textbook of Abdominal Ultrasound. Baltimore: Williams & Wilkins, 1993.

Hagen-Ansert SL: Textbook of Diagnostic Ultrasonography, 3rd ed. St. Louis: C. V. Mosby, 1989

Kremkau FW: Diagnostic Ultrasound: Principles, Instruments, and Exercises, 3rd ed. Philadelphia: W. B. Saunders, 1989.

Mittelstaedt CA: Abdominal Ultrasound. New York: Churchill Livingstone, 1987.

Rumack CM, Wilson SR, Charboneau JW: Diagnostic Ultrasound. St. Louis: C. V. Mosby-Year Book, 1991.

Sarti DA: Diagnostic Ultrasound: Text and Cases, 2nd ed. Chicago: Year Book Medical Publishers, 1987.

Primary Applications of Ultrasound

Abdominal Applications

GALLBLADDER DISEASE

There are few conditions better suited to emergency ultrasound investigation than calculous gallbladder disease. There are many reasons for this, ranging from the anatomic to the demographic. It is incontestable that, in the past decade, real-time sonography of the gallbladder has virtually displaced other investigations as the first step in evaluating this disorder. Although all medical students learn of classic-presentation gallbladder disease, the actual presentation is often nonclassic. The number of patients presenting with epigastric or right upper quadrant pain—which could represent acute cholecystitis—is so great that the emergency physician is fortunate indeed to have at his or her disposal a noninvasive test that ordinarily can confirm or refute the diagnosis with a high degree of accuracy. Although the literature is skewed toward surgical series, it appears that only about one third or less of patients who are suspected of having acute cholecystitis eventually prove to have this diagnosis. Conversely, the significant number of dark-complexioned, nonflatulent, non–40-year-old men who have never had discrete right upper quadrant pain but who are proved to have symptomatic gall-

bladder disease nonetheless is a reminder of the limitations of history and physical examination in making this diagnosis. Although listed for convenience under the rubric "right upper quadrant and epigastric pain," this discussion applies to all cases in which investigation of the gallbladder is warranted by any one of several presenting symptoms. Some patients, for example, complain only of nausea or vomiting; others only have shoulder pain; and some may present frankly septic without the ability to localize the site. Diagnostic emergency ultrasound frequently leads to either a presumptive diagnosis or rapid narrowing of the diagnostic possibilities. When emergency department ultrasound is readily available for such patients, several time-consuming and low-yield investigations may be relegated to an ancillary status or omitted entirely. Plain radiographs of the abdomen and amylase, lipase, and liver function tests are far from obsolete in the evaluation of upper abdominal pain, but their notoriously poor sensitivity and specificity for symptomatic gallbladder disease as compared with "gold standard" right upper quadrant ultrasound has rendered them superfluous in many instances.

General Considerations

The terminology used to refer to symptomatic gallbladder disease is frankly confusing and often ambiguous. Acute cholecystitis and chronic cholecystitis are often used to describe the clinical entities which, at their extremes, are quite distinct. The patient with new onset of upper quadrant pain and tenderness together with a fever and leukocytosis clinically has acute cholecystitis; the patient with a long history of gallstones or recurrent symptomatic bouts of pain has chronic cholecystitis.

Similar clinical distinctions are made for pyelonephritis and pancreatitis. The difficulty is that the pathologic process underlying these various presentations has only a poor correlation with the clinical history. The widespread dissemination of the noninvasive techniques of ultrasound and radionucleotide scanning has allowed both physiologic and anatomic definition of the pathologic condition prior to surgery in almost all cases, and it is sometimes unclear which terminology—the pathologic/radiologic or the clinical—is being used. In addition, gallstones themselves are present in more than 90% of cases of (pathology proved) acute cholecystitis. Conversely, gallstones themselves may be completely asymptomatic with no evidence of "itis" of any type. In any event, symptomatic gallbladder disease clearly represents a broad spectrum of disease that may present to the emergency physician at any clinical or pathologic stage. The great triumph of ultrasound is that it is capable of confirming or refuting gallbladder disease at a very high degree of sensitivity and specificity at any stage in the spectrum. It is fortunate that the vast majority of all symptomatic gallbladder disease (more than 90%) is of the calculus variety. Because ultrasound is exquisitely sensitive in detecting calculi, ultrasound can detect even very tiny gallstones, regardless of their chemical composition.

In all cases, whether calculus or acalculous disease, various signs must be assiduously searched for. These signs are discussed in some detail, because their importance in establishing the gallbladder as a source of the patient's symptoms can hardly be overestimated. Even in the presence of stones, an otherwise negative gallbladder examination would make it highly unlikely that the acute symptomatology is of gallbladder origin. Conversely, even when stones are absent, the presence of these other signs make the diagnosis very likely.

Although ultrasound examination of the gallbladder allows for a confirmed diagnosis in most cases and permits the emergency physician to reach a reasonable disposition in the others, sometimes (particularly with acalculous disease) the ultrasound findings are equivocal or conflict with the clinical impression. The emergency physician must be aware that other means of assessing gallbladder function may well be complementary to ultrasound, and that consultation or referral is required. During the early part of the past decade, there was a collection of articles comparing the relative value of ultrasound and scintigraphy in various acute settings. A consensus has developed that the radionuclide study detects gallbladder function in a way that ultrasound cannot, and is a useful step in those cases where ultrasound is not definitive, and particularly where acute cholecystitis is suspected. It is also a consensus that this subset of patients exists mostly in those with acalculous disease, and that neither study makes that diagnosis reliably. Such patients often require specialized studies by gastroenterology consultants.

Sonographic Considerations of the Gallbladder

"If the gallbladder did not exist, ultrasonographers would have invented it." This statement correctly emphasizes the amazingly favorable characteristics of the gallbladder for ultrasound studies. As Figure 2–1 illustrates, the normal gallbladder is a cystic structure that is filled with an echo-free substance (bile), which is perfectly outlined by the surrounding gallbladder wall. Moreover, the most common sign of gallbladder disease, gallstones themselves, are highly refractile to ultrasound waves. Visualization of calculi of less than 1 mm is routine. In fact, ultrasound may be more sensitive for the detection of stones than either autopsy or operation. Even better for the sonologist is the fact that the whole arrangement is neatly placed under an excellent acoustic window, the liver (as discussed in Chapter 1), which enhances the resolution of ultrasound waves. Figures 2–2 to 2–4 demonstrate the anatomy of the gallbladder in relationship to surrounding structures. With real-time ultrasound, stones are seen to move within the gallbladder. Figure 2–5 shows

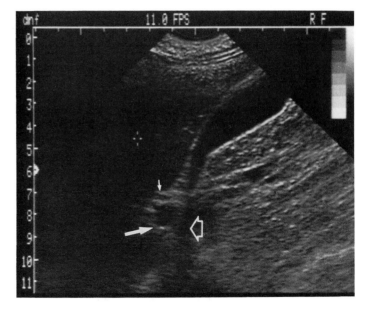

Figure 2-1. Normal gallbladder. This oval, anechoic structure is surrounded by a thin echogenic wall. The common hepatic duct (*small arrow*) is located just anterior to the right portal vein (*large arrow*). The liver lies to the left of the gallbladder in this image. There is acoustic enhancement posterior to the gallbladder, and it is not unusual to see lateral cystic shadowing from the edge of the gallbladder wall (*open arrow*).

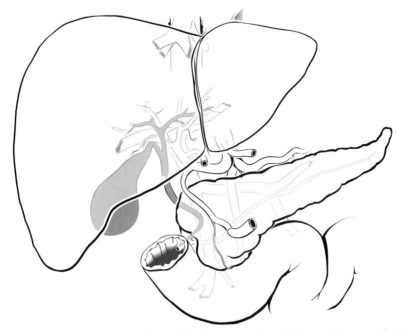

Figure 2-2. Hepatobiliary system. The anatomy of the gallbladder, common hepatic duct, and common bile duct is highlighted (light gray) in relationship to the surrounding anatomy.

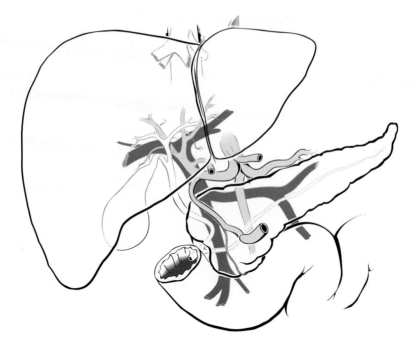

Figure 2–3. Vascular supply to the liver. The anatomy of the celiac axis (light gray), superior mesenteric artery (light gray), and portal venous system (dark gray) is demonstrated in relationship to the surrounding structures. The anatomy of the celiac trunk may be quite variable, but most commonly it branches to form the left gastric, splenic, and hepatic arteries. The splenic and inferior mesenteric veins join the superior mesenteric vein to form the main portal vein.

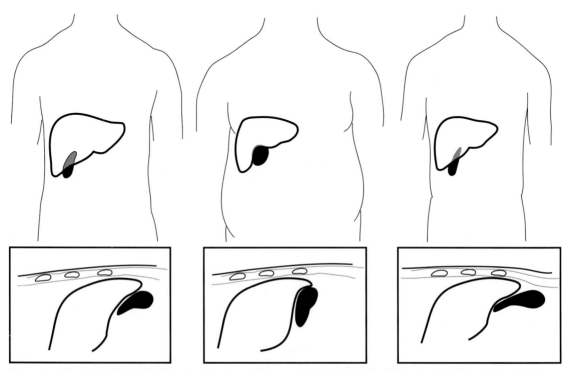

Figure 2–4. Position of the gallbladder. Variations in position occur in individuals with differing body habitus. *Left to right*, location in the normal, obese, and thin patient, respectively.

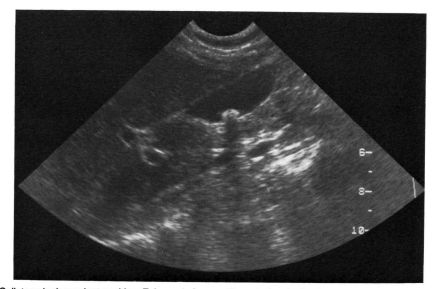

Figure 2–5. Gallstone in dependent position. Echogenic focus with posterior shadowing that moves to dependent position as patient is moved.

a small stone that has moved to a dependent position as the patient's position is changed. Often, blockage of the ultrasound beam by calculi is so prominent that acoustic shadows are easily noted distal to the stones, as can be appreciated in Figures 2–6A–C. It is in fact sometimes easier to see the shadows than the stones themselves. The presence of shadows prompts the sonographer to carefully search in multiple planes for the presence of stones. It is believed that in the majority of cases of acute cholecystitis, symptoms are caused by obstruction of the cystic duct. Movable stones such as those seen in Figure 2–5 are, by definition, not lodged in the duct. Figure 2–7 shows such a stone, which is seen not to move to a dependent position when the patient moves. Stones within the narrow cystic duct can be more difficult to visualize than those in the bile-filled lumen of the gallbladder, and a solitary stone that is passed into the cystic or common duct (Figs. 2–8 to 2–10) may be difficult to directly visualize; in such a situation, secondary findings (particularly focal tenderness) are critical.

Tenderness that is elicited with the probe directly over the gallbladder is referred to as a *sonographic Murphy's sign* (Table 2–1). The sensitivity and specificity of this sign in patients subsequently shown to have acute cholecystitis is approximately 90%. Another very important ultrasound sign is a thickened gallbladder wall,

ordinarily defined as one that measures greater than 3 mm. The gallbladder walls in Figures 2–11 and 2–12, for example, are clearly greater than 3 mm thick and can also be seen to be somewhat multilayered. There is some controversy regarding both the sensitivity and specificity of the thickened wall sign of both acute and chronic cholecystitis. Although it is clearly present in most such patients, gallbladder wall thickening is sometimes seen in edematous states (congestive heart failure, renal failure) and sometimes in the normal post-prandial patient where the gallbladder has recently contracted (Fig. 2–13A and B). Less commonly observed wall abnormalities include the presence of gas that represents emphysematous cholecystitis (see Fig. 1–46A and B) and focal irregularities that may represent microabscess, infarction, or hemorrhage (Fig. 2–14A and B). From the standpoint of the emergency practitioner, it is important only to recognize what an abnormal wall is; the more abnormal it is, the more serious the problem is likely to be. The gallbladder wall shown in Figure 2–14A and B might represent sloughing, hemorrhage, or infection; it is unequivocally abnormal and cause for immediate consultation.

A commonly encountered sonographic finding is that the space within the gallbladder does not appear to be echo-free, but rather exhibits a degree of homogeneous echogenicity that often

Text continued on page 51

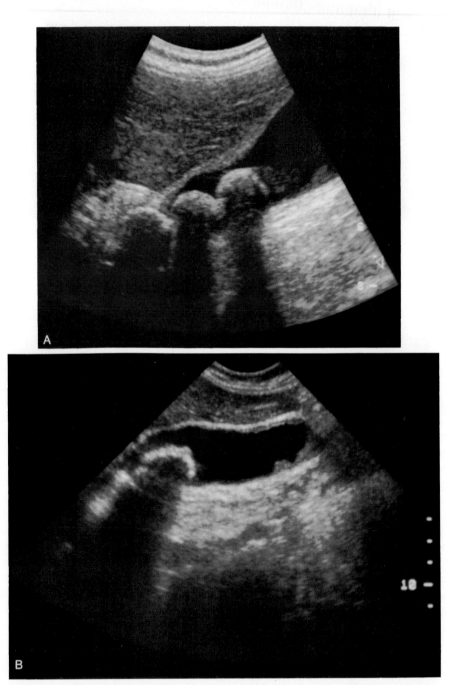

Figure 2–6. Gallstones. *A*, Multiple large gallstones with some wall thickening. *B*, A large gallstone with prominent posterior acoustic shadowing and a small gallstone with minimal shadowing. There is also wall thickening present.

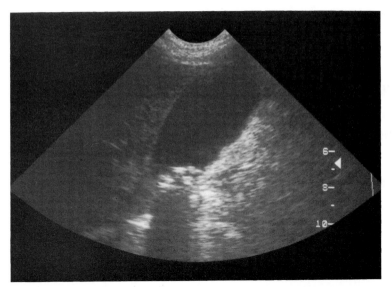

Figure 2-6 *Continued. C*, How multiple small stones shadow as a group.

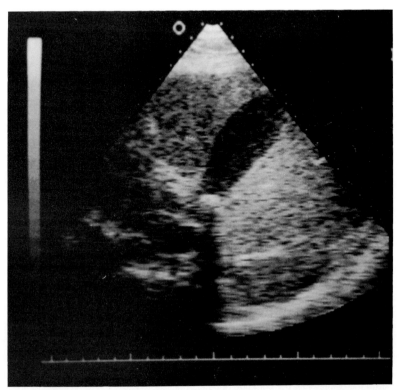

Figure 2-7. Stone in neck of gallbladder. Gallstones that are impacted in the neck of the gallbladder or located in the cystic duct will not move to a dependent position when the patient is moved.

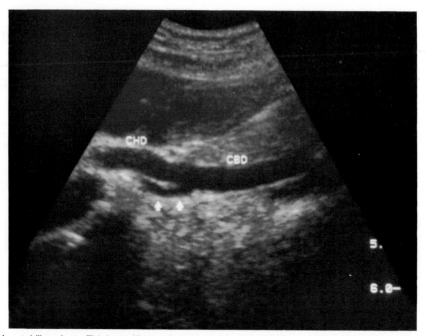

Figure 2–8. Hepatobiliary ducts. This image illustrates the insertion of the cystic duct (*arrows*) into the common hepatic duct to form the common bile duct. Insertion of the cystic duct is often difficult to visualize with ultrasound.

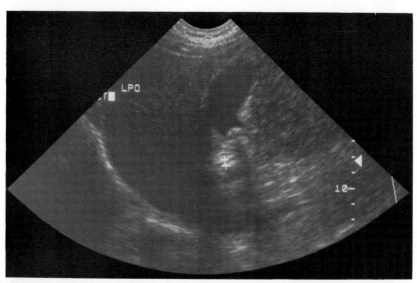

Figure 2–9. Gallstone in cystic duct. This stone is impacted into the neck of the gallbladder at the origin of the cystic duct. The markers demonstrate the diameter of the common hepatic duct.

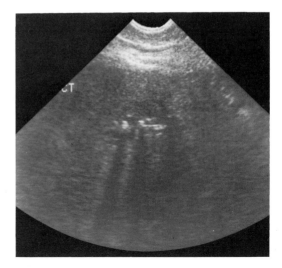

Figure 2-10. Stone in common bile duct. An echogenic focus with posterior shadowing is seen in the common bile duct. These stones are often very difficult to visualize.

Table 2-1. APPROACH TO THE PATIENT WITH ACUTE RIGHT UPPER QUADRANT PAIN

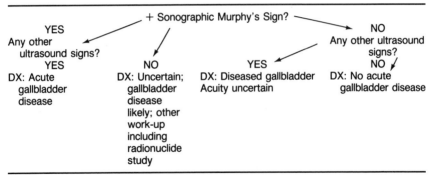

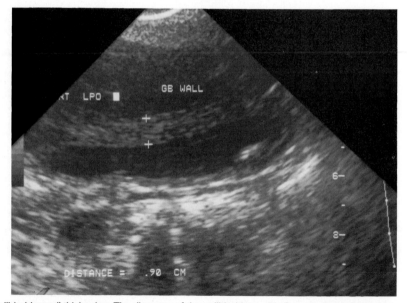

Figure 2–11. Gallbladder wall thickening. The diameter of the gallbladder wall is 9 mm in this patient. A stone is noted in the fundus of the gallbladder. The average wall thicknesses in acute and chronic cholecystitis are 9 mm and 5 mm, respectively; wall thickness is normally ≤3 mm.

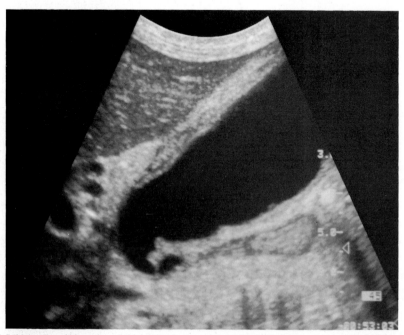

Figure 2–12. Wall thickening. Although wall thickening is associated with cholecystitis, it has also been noted with alcoholic liver disease, ascites, hypoalbuminemia, hepatitis, heart failure, renal failure, and post-prandial state.

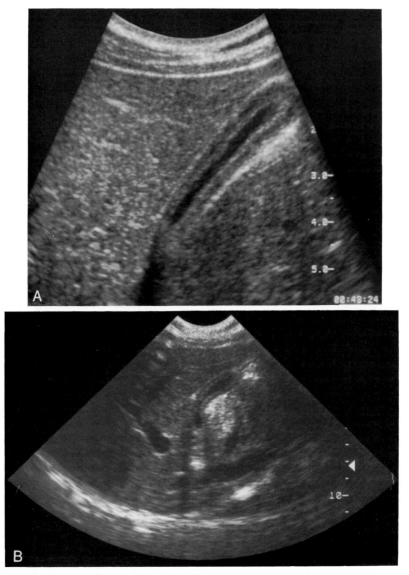

Figure 2 – 13. *A* and *B*, Contracted gallbladder. Approximately two thirds of normal patients completely contract their gallbladder after a fatty meal. The gallbladder remains incompletely contracted in the other one third. The gallbladder wall appears artificially thickened in the contracted state. The contracted gallbladder wall has a reflective outer and inner contour, with an anechoic region between these two layers.

approaches that of the surrounding liver. This material can be seen in Figures 2 – 15 to 2 – 18 in the dependent position and is commonly referred to as "sludge." Sludge represents echogenic bile, related to stasis; the clinical significance of sludge is difficult to deduce from the literature. Sludge is quite common in acute cholecystitis (about 50% of cases have it), but it is also seen in conditions of fasting and is common with nursing home patients with poor oral intake. Sludge is not usually found in ambulatory

patients; its presence in this setting is highly suggestive, perhaps diagnostic of gallbladder disease. Sludge may take several minutes to assume a dependent position.

Although the gallbladder is among the easiest of all organs to visualize, caveats are in order. The procedure is performed with either the 3.5- or the 5-MHz probe. Many sonographers begin the examination just under the right costal margin in the mid-clavicular line. The supine position is usually perfectly satisfac-

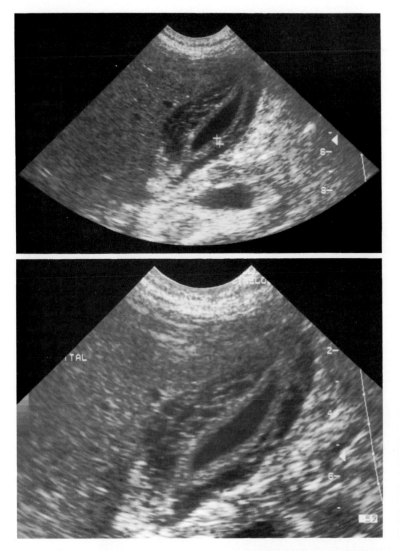

Figure 2–14. *A* and *B*, Septated pericholecystic fluid. This appearance may represent abscess, infarction, or hemorrhage into or around the gallbladder wall. These images were obtained from a patient with human immunodeficiency virus (HIV) disease. Cytomegalovirus (CMV) and cryptosporidium infections are associated with acalculous inflammation of the biliary tract.

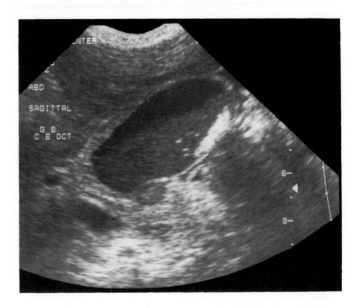

Figure 2–15. Sludge. This image demonstrates sludge and multiple gallstones within the gallbladder.

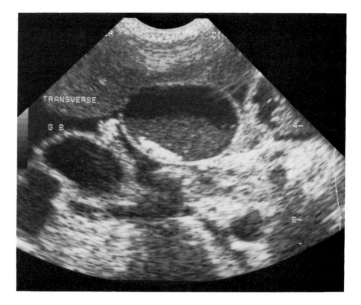

Figure 2–16. Sludge. There are echogenic bile (sludge) and multiple bright echogenic foci with posterior shadowing (stones) within the gallbladder. In addition, there is free ascitic fluid surrounding the gallbladder.

tory with the patient moved to the left posterior oblique position (Fig. 2–19) in order to demonstrate the mobility of calculi or sludge. Standing the patient upright is often a good method to demonstrate stones and sludge. The gallbladder moves remarkably with respiration; it is often convenient to use this respiratory excursion as a way of scanning through the organ at different levels. Frequently, visualization is maximized by positioning the probe in an intercostal space, which has the advantages of avoiding interfer-

ence with bowel gas and causing less discomfort to the patient. The gallbladder is identified and is examined in the long and the short axis, special care being taken to attempt visualization of the neck of the gallbladder, where, as mentioned, an obstructing stone is likely to be found. The main lobar fissure of the liver (a linear echogenic structure) points toward the gallbladder neck in the sagittal section (Figures 2–20 and 2–21). Some sonologists find this useful. The absolute dimensions of the gallbladder are

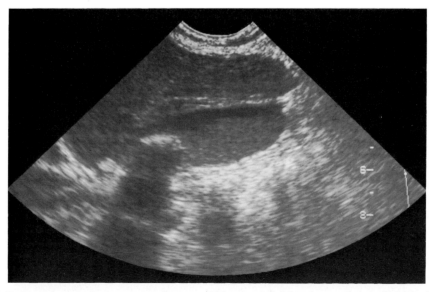

Figure 2–17. Sludge and stones. In contrast to gallstones, which generate bright echoes and acoustic shadowing, sludge exhibits low to moderate level echoes without acoustic shadowing.

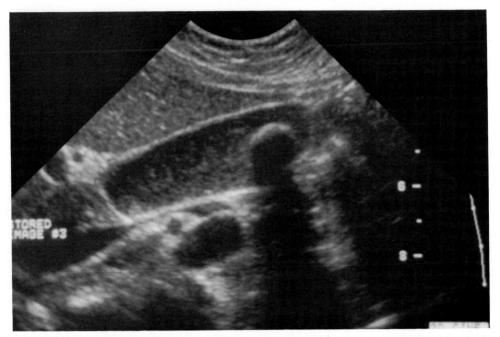

Figure 2–18. Sludge associated with a large gallstone. Sludge is very viscous; thus, it moves slowly after the patient is repositioned.

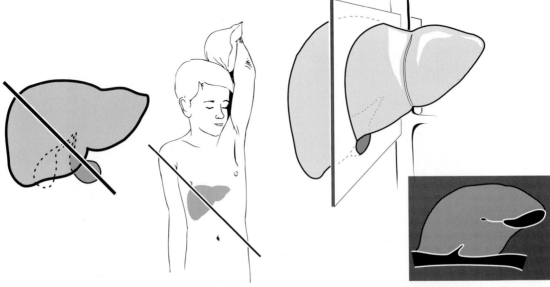

Figure 2–19. Left posterior oblique. Placing the patient into this position (also referred to as oblique right-side-up position) allows the sonographer to demonstrate mobility of gallstones. In addition, scanning of the common bile duct is more easily performed in this position.

Figure 2–20. Middle hepatic plane. One can often identify the main lobar fissure as a linear echogenic structure that connects the neck of the gallbladder with the right portal vein. The middle hepatic vein is seen entering the inferior vena cava in the cross-sectional view.

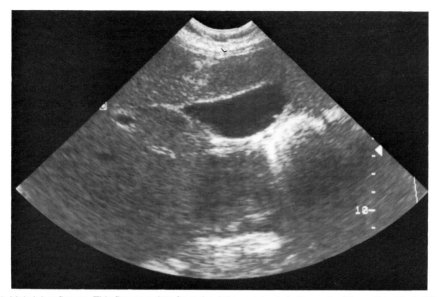

Figure 2–21. Main lobar fissure. This fissure points from the right portal vein to the neck of the gallbladder in this sagittal section.

not of critical importance: "normals" have been listed up to 11 to 13 cm (Fig. 2–22). Without any other signs, the large gallbladder, like the very small gallbladder, more likely represents the state of alimentation rather than anything else. The large, very tender gallbladder raises the suspicion of obstruction; in that situation, size could have considerable importance.

Although emergency physicians do not have the luxury of preparing their patients with a 6-hour fast, most patients with symptomatic gallbladder disease will not have recently eaten voraciously. When ultrasound examinations are performed on patients with mild symptoms, especially those with epigastric rather than right upper quadrant pain, a significant number (between 5 and 10% of emergency department examinations will be unsuccessful due simply to the contracted state of the post-prandial gallbladder (congenital absence is said to afflict

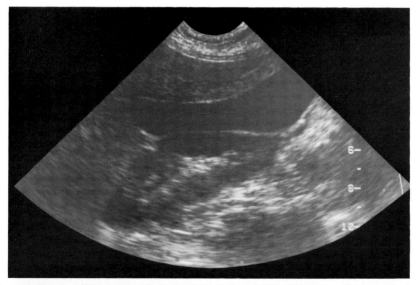

Figure 2–22. Large gallbladder. This usually reflects the state of alimentation rather than a disease entity; however, a large, tender gallbladder suggests the possibility of obstruction.

0.03% of the population). The ability of rare patients to eat whole meals while being worked up in the emergency department for pain, nausea, and vomiting cannot be dismissed lightly. The typical post-prandial scan, shown in Figure 2–13A and B, shows the gallbladder to be slightly more than 1 cm in diameter and could easily be mistaken for a vessel cut in cross section. In a contracted state, the gallbladder wall can be expected to appear *thickened* when it has no pathologic change.

The shape of the gallbladder is often mentioned as a secondary sign of disease, but there seems to be a significant subjective component to the evaluation. The normal gallbladder is pear shaped, tapering down gracefully to the neck. Many gallbladders, however, have a somewhat irregular shape; a commonly encountered variant is referred to as the *phrygian cap* (Fig. 2–23A and B). Other common variants include septa (either complete or incomplete) or junctional folds extending from the gallbladder wall, as in Figure 2–24, or the presence of very prominent spiral valves in the neck of the gallbladder (Fig. 2–25), which can look very strikingly like an impacted stone. Careful examina-

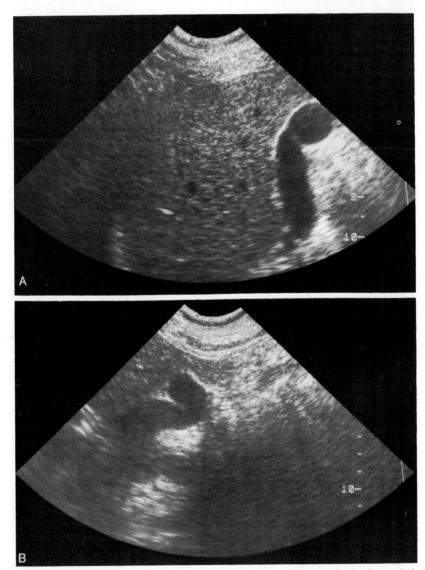

Figure 2–23. *A* and *B*, Phrygian cap. This is a fold of the distal segment of the gallbladder that is of no pathologic significance; it is seen in approximately 4% of the population.

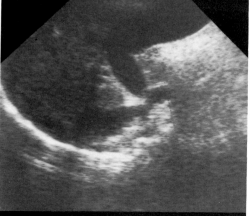

Figure 2–24. Junctional fold. This occurs most commonly between the body and the infundibulum, as is demonstrated in this image. Folds, caps, or kinks in the gallbladder are noted in approximately 15% of normal patients.

tion reveals that although more reflective than expected, the valve does not have the same reflectivity as do calculi and does not cast acoustic shadows.

There are, of course, many conditions and variants that can cause confusion even to the ex-

perienced sonographer. Relatively few occur with frequency, and fewer still are likely to be interpreted as normal when they are not. One easily missed abnormality has already been mentioned: the stone impacted in the cystic duct (Figs. 2–7 and 2–9). The second situation that deserves special attention is that of the patient with long-standing gallbladder disease in whom the gallbladder is scarred down, surrounding a nucleus of calculi. It might first be thought that this would present an obvious appearance (indeed, these are the types of cases where stones can often be seen on plain radiographs), but the ultrasound appearance may in fact be extremely difficult to interpret. Because the scarred gallbladder is contracted to fit tightly over the stones, there is little or no remaining lumen and often no bile at all. Thus, the usual appearance is radically altered; all that remains is a hyperechoic area, perhaps with distal shadowing, but without any of the familiar gallbladder landmarks (Figs. 1–43A and 2–26). This situation should be considered whenever the gallbladder cannot be located, particularly if there is a suspicion of long-standing disease. Another quite different cause of error is the so-called pseudo sludge phenomenon. This common artifact mimicks sludge

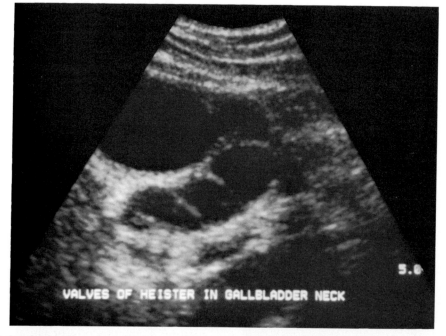

Figure 2–25. Spiral valves. The valves of Heister can be seen in the neck of the gallbladder as echogenic protrusions that do not shadow.

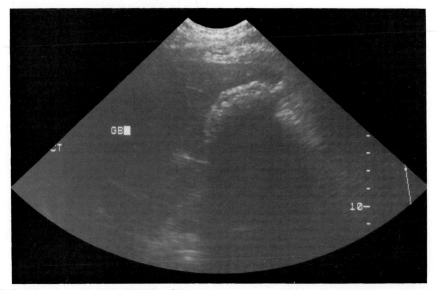

Figure 2–26. Stones in a contracted gallbladder. Gallstones may prevent ultrasound visualization of the gallbladder. This image demonstrates the double arc or WES triad (wall, echo, shadow). The proximal arc is the wall of the gallbladder, followed by the anechoic bile above the echogenic stones, which cast prominent posterior shadows.

within the bladder lumen. This is shown in Figure 1–49 and is best appreciated during real-time scanning. The cause of this artifact is technical (see Chapter 1), but this pseudo sludge often can be seen to extend beyond the gallbladder walls. Figures 2–27 to 2–32 illustrate some unusual sonographic findings, including septated gallstones, comet-tail shadowing from cholesterol stones, cholesterosis of the gallbladder, floating gallstones, and a gallbladder mass.

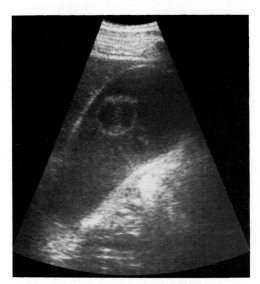

Figure 2–27. Septated gallstone.

Clinical Considerations

As with much of emergency ultrasound, selection of patients for gallbladder ultrasound varies greatly according to availability of appropriate equipment, personnel, and local practice. There is little question, however, that emergency use will increase greatly as a result of incorporation of ultrasound as an integral part of emergency medicine practice and the conviction that such technologies should be available to symptomatic emergency department patients at all times of the day and week. One extreme would be to reserve right upper quadrant ultrasound strictly to those emergency department patients who have clinical conditions such that delayed performance of the examination is likely to increase morbidity/mortality significantly. Even this conservative standard is not currently met in many emergency departments, where scanning is simply unavailable outside of standard business hours. The opposing view would be to use ultrasound where it is likely to be of benefit to the diagnosis, treatment, or disposition of the emergency department patient; that is, it should be used according to the same principles that govern the use of direct laryngoscopy, sigmoidoscopy, or slit-lamp examination. In each of these cases, the particular examination is conducted when the emergency

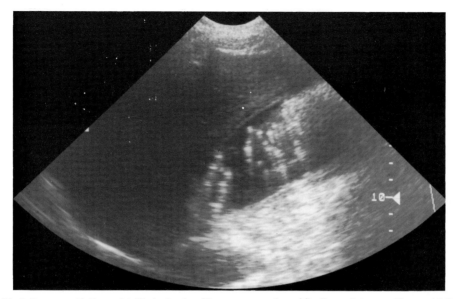

Figure 2–28. Gallstones with "comet-tail" shadowing. There are a number of floating gallstones with comet-tail shadowing present in this image. This pattern occurs more commonly with cholesterol stones. In addition, there is prominent wall thickening in this patient with acute cholecystitis.

physician judges that the patient is likely to gain significant benefit from the procedure. In some institutions where ultrasound has been incorporated into daily practice, emergency physicians believe that their examinations of patients with epigastric and particularly right upper quadrant pain are incomplete without sonographic visualization of the gallbladder.

Evidence has already appeared, both domestically and abroad, to indicate that emergency ultrasound examination of the right upper quadrant can be performed with accuracy similar to that of traditional ultrasound specialists. In this early stage of rapid change, perhaps some guidelines can be initiated. At the very least, ultrasound of the right upper quadrant

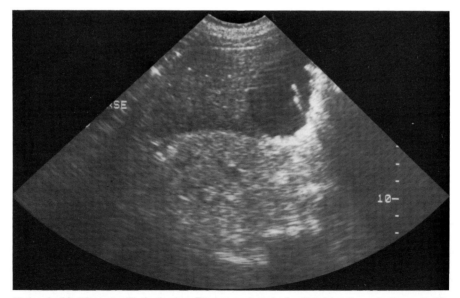

Figure 2–29. "Comet-tail" shadowing. Transverse image of gallbladder shown in Figure 2–28.

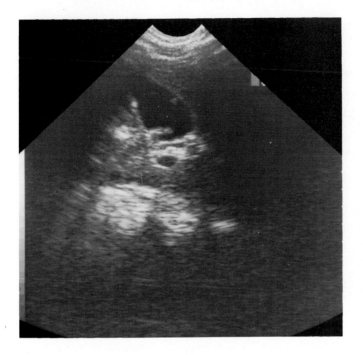

Figure 2–30. Cholesterosis of the gallbladder. Cholesterol polyps are attached to the friable mucosa of the gallbladder wall. These echogenic masses occasionally can have posterior acoustic shadowing, and thus may be confused with gallstones. In contrast to gallstones, these structures remain attached to the gallbladder wall with changes in the patient's position.

should be promptly available (within an hour) for emergency department patients when the clinical presentation is such that delay in confirmation or refutation of diagnosis of acute gallbladder disease would be likely to significantly increase their morbidity. An example of how this might be applied is the septic elderly patient who presents with fever, chills, and abdominal pain from an undetermined cause. Antibiotics will be started in any case, and documentation of a biliary rather than a urinary source would allow not only for rational antibiotic therapy, but also for early surgical consultation. Another example might be the juvenile-onset diabetic

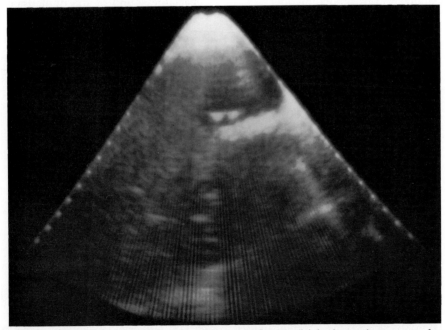

Figure 2–31. Floating stones. This image demonstrates two stones floating slightly above a large group of smaller stones (gravel) that cast a prominent posterior shadow. Floating stones are more commonly cholesterol or gas-containing stones.

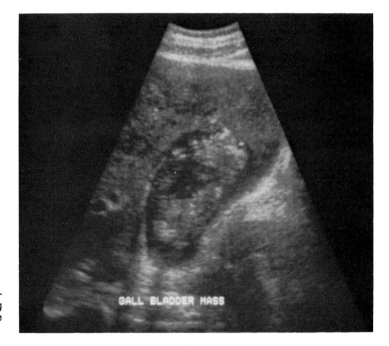

Figure 2–32. Gallbladder mass. This ultrasound appearance of a mass filling the gallbladder lumen is very suggestive of carcinoma of the gallbladder.

with gallbladder disease who presents with right upper quadrant pain, fever, and perhaps acidosis. A confirmed ultrasound diagnosis of gangrenous cholecystitis (Fig. 2-33A – C) or gallbladder perforation (occurring in 8 to 12% of patients with acute cholecystitis) facilitates the correct medical and surgical approach to such a critical problem.

A moderate, middle-of-the-road standard dictates that right upper quadrant ultrasound promptly be performed on emergency departments patients in whom delay in confirmation or refutation of the diagnosis will result in a significant delay in instituting appropriate treatment, arranging for appropriate disposition, or whose discomfort would be significantly increased or prolonged by delayed evaluation. An example is the young woman with persistent right-sided abdominal pain and leukocytosis: in such a case, the differential diagnosis might well include acute cholecystitis and acute appendicitis. Prompt right upper quadrant ultrasound in such patients is likely to be of significant benefit in at least two ways. If the diagnosis of acute cholecystitis is confirmed, the patient could be treated with potent narcotic analgesics, as well as with appropriate antibiotics. In most institutions, analgesics would not be provided to such patients while the diagnosis was uncer-

tain and observation for appendicitis was ongoing. Also, if right upper quadrant ultrasound refuted the diagnosis of acute cholecystitis, the possibility of appendicitis would be correspondingly greater. It is likely that earlier operative intervention would then be justified.

A third approach would be to use ultrasound examination of the gallbladder in all patients to whom it would be likely to provide a clinical benefit in terms of hastening the diagnosis of symptomatic gallbladder disease or shortening the time required for the investigation of other possible problems. For example, the classic 40-year-old, flatulent woman with recurrent abdominal distress who was not acutely ill would fall into this category. Immediate ultrasound examination confirms the diagnosis during the one visit to the emergency department and avoids the necessity of performing other, less specific tests. Referral to an appropriate source for definitive therapy is simplified.

Summary of Positive Findings

Ultrasound examination of the gallbladder is, in a sense, more complex than the other primary studies because there are a number of possible positive findings, which may occur in any possible combination. Conversely, these findings are usually very easy to recognize.

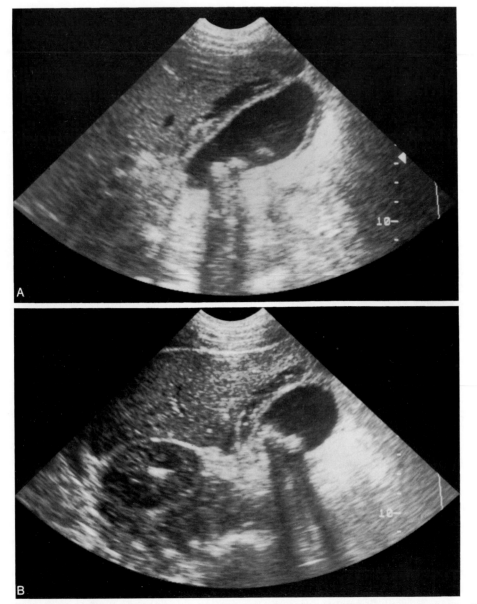

Figure 2–33. Gangrenous cholecystitis. Striations in the gallbladder wall are the most common ultrasound finding of this disorder. The sagittal (*A*) and transverse (*B*) scans demonstrate multiple gallstones within the gallbladder and significant wall thickening.

It is important to search diligently for the principal and ancillary sonographic signs; it is, however, even more important to remember that the most important finding is *tenderness to probe pressure*. Without this sonographic Murphy's sign, the diagnosis of gallbladder disease as *a cause of the patient's acute symptoms* is always in doubt. Conversely, when the sign is clearly present, even in the absence of other findings, symptomatic gallbladder disease is likely.

The two other principal findings, *gallstones* (Figs. 2–34 to 2–38) and *wall abnormalities* (usually pathologic thickening), are diagnostic of gallbladder disease, but either finding by itself does not prove that gallbladder disease is the cause of ongoing symptoms. In general, focal tenderness with any other principal or ancillary sign (such as sludge, pericholecystic fluid, a clearly abnormal size or shape) makes the diagnosis of acute gallbladder disease with greater—sometimes much greater—than 90%

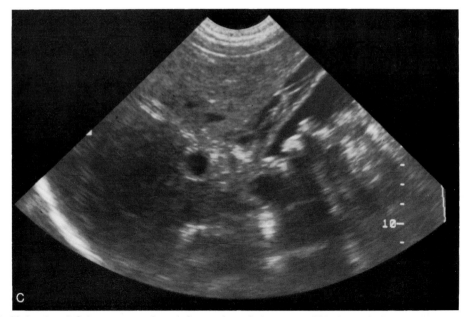

Figure 2–33 *Continued.* C demonstrates the striations and anechoic spaces within the markedly thickened gallbladder wall.

certainty. Table 2–2 summarizes focal tenderness combinations in the diagnosis of acute gallbladder disease.

Clearly, in the patient who is not currently symptomatic, tenderness is much less likely to be found and its absence means less. In such a case, any two of the principal or ancillary signs make gallbladder disease as a cause of recent symptoms likely.

Finally, in an acutely symptomatic patient in whom the diagnosis is uncertain (scenarios 2 or 3), radionuclide scanning usually resolves the issue. If the gallbladder does not visualize in this patient, cholecystitis is very likely. In addition, if emptying does not occur in response to an appropriate stimulus (e.g., a fatty meal), an obstructed duct is likely. If visualization and emptying are normal, it is unlikely that acute

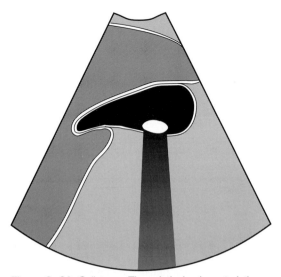

Figure 2–34. Gallstone. The relatively characteristic appearance of a gallstone within the gallbladder, demonstrating an echogenic structure with posterior shadowing.

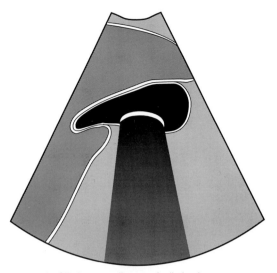

Figure 2–35. Large gallstone. A distinctive appearance, where there are echoes originating only from the anterior surface of the stone, producing a crescent shape with posterior shadowing.

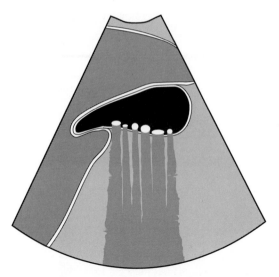

Figure 2-36. Multiple smaller stones. The typical appearance with multiple echogenic foci with indistinct shadowing.

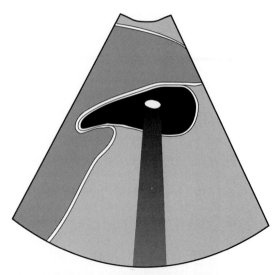

Figure 2-37. Floating gallstone. Stone in the upper lumen of the gallbladder with strong posterior shadowing. Floating gallstones are more likely to be cholesterol stones with a significantly lower calcium content. Gas-containing stones have also been described to float.

gallbladder disease is present. In particular circumstances, where the point of tenderness is not certain or a question of duct dilatation exists, computed tomography (CT) may be a reasonable option.

Common Errors in Gallbladder Scanning

1. Failure to use the decubitus, "belly out," and erect positions when evaluating possible stones or sludge
2. Misdiagnosis of a hyperechoic spiral valve as an impacted stone
3. Failure to identify an impacted stone at the neck of the gallbladder
4. Overdiagnosing gallbladder wall thickness in the post-prandial patient or in the patient with edema

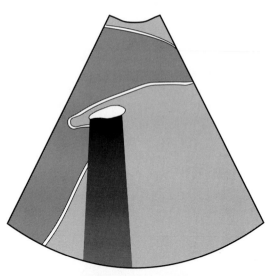

Figure 2-38. Contracted gallbladder. Appears as an echogenic focus (filled with stones) with posterior shadowing. The lumen of the gallbladder is not visualized in this setting. The ultrasound appearance of the duodenum may occasionally mimic a contracted gallbladder that is filled with stones.

Table 2-2. FOCAL TENDERNESS COMBINATIONS IN THE DIAGNOSIS OF GALLBLADDER DISEASE

This sign	Plus any
1. +Focal tenderness	+abnormal wall +stones +sludge } = acute gallbladder disease +abnormal size +abnormal shape
2. +Focal tenderness	+no other signs present = acute gallbladder disease likely; further work-up indicated
3. −Focal tenderness	+any combination = gallbladder disease likely or definite, acute disease uncertain, further work-up
4. −Focal tenderness	+no other signs = no gallbladder disease

5. Diagnosing artifacts in the gallbladder as sludge

6. Incomplete visualization of the gallbladder fundus from failure to use the intercostal approach

7. Failure to correctly identify the gallbladder when it looks atypically hyperechoic due to multiple stones and little bile

8. Mistaking the normal artifact generated at the gallbladder edges for acoustic shadowing caused by stones

9. Not visualizing the entire gallbladder lumen because it is folded over

10. Missing very small stones when they do not cause shadows

SELECTED READINGS

Gallbladder Disease

Engel JM, Deitch EA, Sikkema W: Gallbladder wall thickness: Sonographic accuracy and relation to disease. AJR 1980;134:907–909.

Laing FC: Diagnostic evaluation of patients with suspected acute cholecystitis. Radiol Clin North Am 1983;21:477–493.

Marchal G, Van de Voorde P, Van Dooren W, et al: Ultrasonic appearance of the filled and contracted normal gallbladder. J Clin Ultrasound 1980;8:439–442.

Marton KI, Doubilet P: How to image the gallbladder in suspected cholecystitis. Ann Intern Med 1988;109:722–729.

Mirvis SE, Vainright JR, Nelson AW, et al: The diagnosis of acute calculous cholecystitis: A comparison of sonography, scintigraphy, and CT. AJR 1986;147:1171–1175.

Nemcek AA, Gore RM, Vogelzang RL, Grant M: The effervescent gallbladder: A sonographic sign of emphysematous cholecystitis. AJR 1988;150:575–577.

Ralls PW, Colletti PM, Lapin SA, et al: Real-time sonography in suspected acute cholecystitis: Prospective evaluation of primary and secondary signs. Radiology 1985;155:767–771.

Ralls PW, Quinn MF, Juttner HU, et al: Gallbladder wall thickening: Patients without intrinsic gallbladder disease. AJR 1981;137:65–68.

OBSTRUCTIVE UROPATHY

Renal colic is the form of acute obstructive uropathy most commonly seen by emergency physicians. This problem is viewed somewhat differently by emergency physicians than by practitioners of other specialties, to whom the diagnosis may seem rather mundane. It is, after all, not ordinarily a life-threatening diagnosis; the diagnosis is often straightforward; and treatment for the acute event has changed little in several decades. In many respects, however, it represents an emergency medicine problem par excellence. First and most obviously, the condition is extremely ubiquitous: at least 15%

of all American males will suffer a stone event that requires emergent medical attention. In busy emergency departments, it is not uncommon to have multiple patients who suffer from renal colic in the department simultaneously. Renal colic presents the emergency physician with a series of decisions, including confirmation of the diagnosis, institution of therapy, and disposition, all of which may vary according to institutional practice and all of which are designed to relieve the patient from the extreme pain that has been noted since at least the time of Hippocrates. Emergency ultrasound can often play a key and, occasionally, an indispensable role in effecting this goal.

Diagnostic Considerations

In the most straightforward case of a patient with previous episodes of renal colic who presents with flank pain and hematuria, there is often no need for any imaging procedure at all. Prompt initiation of potent analgesic and perhaps antiprostaglandin therapy proceeds immediately. Response to this therapy, marked by prolonged resolution of pain, is often appropriately used as a guide to the physician that expectant management is indicated. The patient may pass the stone in the emergency department or, more commonly, can be discharged on an oral regimen with the expectation that the offending stone will be passed in an outpatient setting. Although plain radiographs (kidney, ureter, bladder) were once routinely obtained in such patients, recent investigations have indicated that these radiographs add little to the management of renal colic. Because the severe pain of ureteral colic is caused mostly by obstruction and distention of the more proximal urinary collecting system, persistent resolution of the pain is taken as a clinical indicator that high-grade obstruction does not exist. It is for this reason that rapid and cost-effective management of such patients is possible and rational without direct visualization of either the stone or the degree of distention of the urinary system.

Unfortunately, there are a great number of situations, some of them very common, in which direct imaging of the urinary tract is necessary or desirable either to confirm the diagnosis or to allow proper disposition. In these cases, the emergency physician must make a choice between intravenous pyelography (IVP) or diagnostic ultrasound. Several studies have directly compared the two techniques in terms of sensitivity and specificity; all have confirmed that both procedures are very useful and most have found IVP somewhat more specific. Such overall comparisons are of little use to the physician treating an individual patient; what is more important is that each imaging procedure has its own particular strengths and efficiencies that make it the procedure of choice for a given case.

The benefits and advantages to IVP are familiar to most physicians. IVP has long been the gold standard for diagnosing acute ureteral colic; in the past, IVP was alleged to have beneficial properties in promoting passage of the stone (this has never been shown). IVP ordinarily gives excellent visualization of the collecting system and allows for identification of the site of obstruction, usually allowing for identification of the obstructing stone itself. In addition, extravasation of contrast into the retroperitoneal space may be demonstrated, thus confirming high-grade obstruction; this finding itself is used in some centers as one criterion for admission. Other abnormalities of the kidney and collecting system, both congenital and acquired, are often identified by IVP (these include cysts, renal masses, duplications of the collecting system, abnormal size, shape, and location of the kidneys, etc.) and may be of clinical importance. The disadvantages of IVP are considerably more relevant to the emergency physician than they are to those managing patients in the inpatient setting. It is precisely these disadvantages that make ultrasound examinations (often bedside ultrasound) such an attractive option for many emergency patients. Table 2–3 lists some of these all too practical problems.

Table 2–3. CONDITIONS IN WHICH ULTRASOUND MAY BE PREFERABLE TO INTRAVENOUS PYELOGRAPHY

Pregnancy
Contrast allergy
Diabetes mellitus
Proteinuria
Renal failure
Dehydration
Poor venous access
Differential diagnosis includes gallbladder, appendix, pelvic inflammatory disease
Time constraints

The question of availability varies greatly according to institution. In many emergency departments, the emergency physician is able to administer the contrast him- or herself while the x-ray technician takes the plain radiographs required. In places where this is limited either by custom, regulation, or staffing considerations, IVP is effectively unavailable or available only after considerable delay during many hours of the week. Even when the ability to obtain IVP is continually available, many radiology departments insist on documentation of renal function by obtaining a blood urea nitrogen (BUN) or creatine titer prior to the IVP study. This too has the effect of significantly increasing the time (as well as the cost) of the procedure. In addition, the familiar hazards of giving contrast to patients who may be dehydrated or who have proteinuria, diabetes mellitus, or congestive failure are often very real concerns. The question of pregnancy also must be addressed prior to obtaining an IVP, as must a history of previous allergies to contrast and perhaps shellfish, which further impairs the applicability of IVP. To the urologist working up a patient in the hospital, almost all these concerns can be obviated: hydration, correction of congestive failure, control of diabetes, elucidation of possible past allergies, pretreatment with steroids and antihistamines, and use of nonionic contrast material are all options that are less applicable to the busy emergency physician.

Ultrasound examination, although less sensitive for demonstrating small stones, particularly in the distal ureter, does avoid all of the stated disadvantages of IVP, although it does not give an indication of renal function itself. What ultrasound can do, usually very quickly, is demonstrate the results of an obstructing stone: hydroureter and hydronephrosis. As with so many uses of emergency ultrasound, the emergency department examination for suspected renal colic is best viewed as a highly focused study: the confirmation or refutation of significant obstructive uropathy based on the presence or absence of proximal dilatation.

It is debatable which study, IVP or ultrasound, is more sensitive in demonstrating obstruction; i.e., which one should be the gold standard. One study showed ultrasound to be 100% accurate in diagnosing "moderate to severe" hydronephrosis. It is stated that a brisk, intravenously induced diuresis may be overinterpreted on ultrasound as hydroureter; conversely, significant dehydration, especially during this first hour of symptoms, may prevent dilatation from being seen. It should, however, be noted that there are certain rather common abnormalities for which ultrasound is unsurpassed. This is particularly true with the identification of renal cysts and the differentiation of renal masses as being solid or cystic. These are not uncommonly found in the course of emergency department ultrasound examinations and are, at times, of clinical significance.

Sonographic Considerations of the Kidney

There are several factors that make renal ultrasound, particularly for the limited purpose described previously, rather rapid and straightforward when performed either in the radiology suite or at the bedside. First, although no real preparation is necessary, it is true that the markedly dehydrated patient will diurese less than normal and that mild degrees of obstruction will be more difficult to note in such a patient. Basic principles of good medical care, as well as the desire to obtain useful information from the ultrasound, dictate that such a patient receive intravenous hydration. Anatomic considerations make the right kidney more accessible to ultrasound than the left kidney; virtually all right kidneys can be rather easily visualized. Ultrasound examination of the left kidney is hampered by the lack of the overlying liver—which acts as an excellent acoustic window—on the right, as well as by the air-filled stomach, which often hampers optimal scanning anteriorly to the left. Dilated loops of bowel often present a problem, especially on the left, but this can almost always be circumvented by finding another, often more posterior, window. Most commonly, scanning is done intercostally from the lateral approach, using the liver as an acoustic window on the right and the spleen as a window on the left. The 3.5-MHz transducer is ordinarily used in adults, although very good images can often be obtained in thin subjects with the 5-MHz probe. Most beginning sonologists are surprised at the great mobility—2.5 cm with respiration—that the kidneys demonstrate.

The normal appearance of the kidney is quite distinctive, and the organ is among the easiest to recognize. In long section (Fig. 2–39A), the kidney has a football-shaped appearance with a clearly demarcated renal cortex that appears brighter (more reflective), at times referred to as a thick, jagged stripe going down the length of the football-shaped organ. The reason for this appearance may not be obvious at first; it is due to the fact that the tissue that makes up the collecting system has more fat and is therefore more reflective than is the tissue of the renal medulla. It is fortunate that collecting system tissue is more sonodense: it makes dilatation of the collecting system by fluid (echo free) very obvious. When seen in cross sections (short-axis view), the kidney appears C-shaped and again the collecting system is easily visualized as the brighter structure in the center (Fig. 2–39B). A duplicated collecting system is a normal variant (Fig. 2–40) that should not be confused with a pathologic process.

The brighter area surrounding the kidney represents Gerota's fascia and the associated perinephric fat. This abuts Glisson's capsule on the right, covering the liver, and creates an excellent area to look sonographically for intraperitoneal fluid. As one might predict (Fig. 2–41), this fluid appears as an echo-free black space between the two coverings. Figure 2–42 illustrates the commonly encountered difficulty of overlying hepatic or splenic flexure obscuring visualization of the entire kidney. Figure 2–43 shows the same patient as in Figure 2–42, in which the transducer was moved more posteriorly (to the posterior axillary line), now permitting a complete scan. The kidney is traditionally measured in its longest axis; the two kidneys are ordinarily 9 to 12 cm in length, 4 to 5 cm in width, and within 2 cm of each other in terms of size. A difference greater than this can be the result of chronic renal disease that causes the affected kidney to be smaller or acute inflammation or infection that causes the affected kidney to be larger. In some patients, the renal pyramids are surprisingly hypoechoic and prominent; they should not be mistaken for cysts. Figures 2–44 to 2–46 show the anatomic structure of the kidney and organs adjacent to the kidneys.

Although much ancillary information can be gained through complete renal scanning, the focus of the bedside examination of the patient

Text continued on page 72

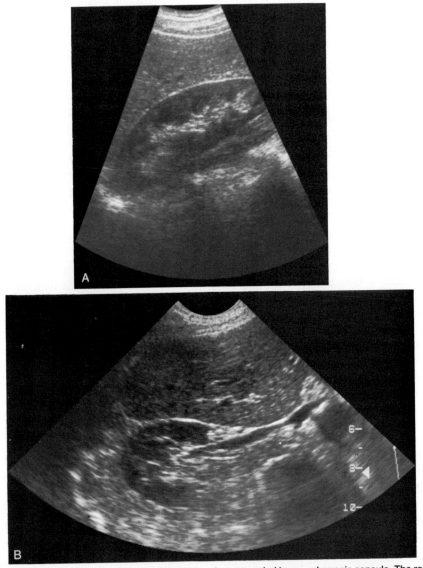

Figure 2–39. *A*, Longitudinal view of normal kidney. The kidney is surrounded by an echogenic capsule. The renal cortex is slightly less echogenic than the adjacent liver, and the renal medulla appears as hypoechoic areas that point to the center of the kidney. The central region is the renal sinus. *B*, Transverse view of normal kidney. The kidney appears C-shaped in cross section, and the renal vein is easier to visualize secondary to its anterior position in comparison to the renal artery. The liver is immediately above the right kidney in this view.

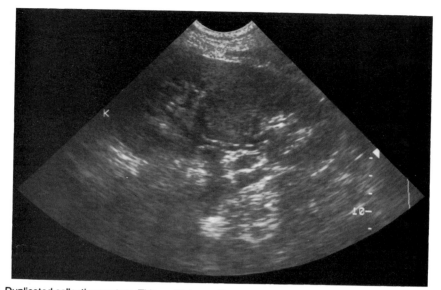

Figure 2-40. Duplicated collecting system. This sagittal scan illustrates two echo-dense regions in the center of the kidney.

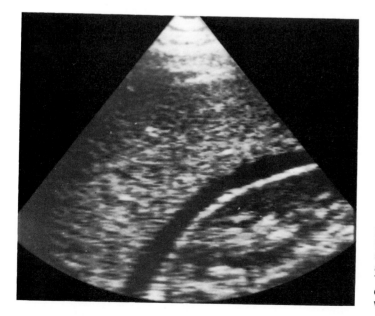

Figure 2-41. Fluid in Morison's pouch. Morison's pouch is normally a potential space between Glisson's capsule of the liver and Gerota's fascia surrounding the kidney. This ultrasound image demonstrates an anechoic stripe above the kidney in a patient with intraperitoneal hemorrhage.

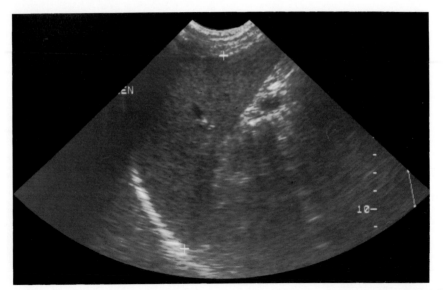

Figure 2–42. Gas in splenic flexure. This is a common finding that interferes with visualization of the left kidney.

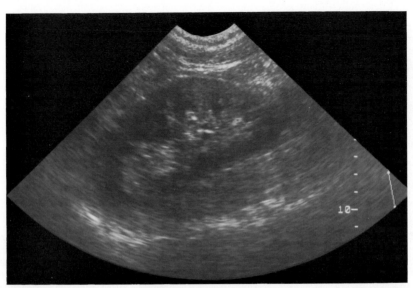

Figure 2–43. Normal left kidney. This is the same patient that was imaged in Figure 2–42; however, the transducer was moved posteriorly, allowing for visualization of the entire left kidney.

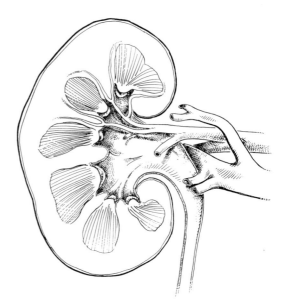

Figure 2–44. Normal kidney. A schematic drawing of the right kidney with the right renal vein seen anterior to the renal artery. The renal medulla forms the pyramids that point toward the pelvis of the kidney. The renal cortex has a homogeneous appearance on ultrasound, which is slightly less echogenic than the neighboring liver. The medulla is significantly less echogenic than the surrounding cortex. The renal pelvis appears as an echogenic central complex within the kidney.

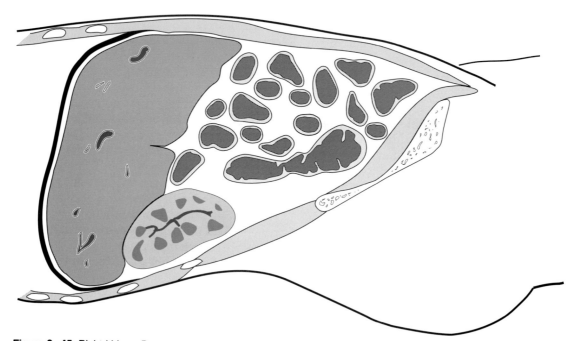

Figure 2–45. Right kidney. Demonstrates a longitudinal section of the right kidney and the surrounding organs (liver and bowel).

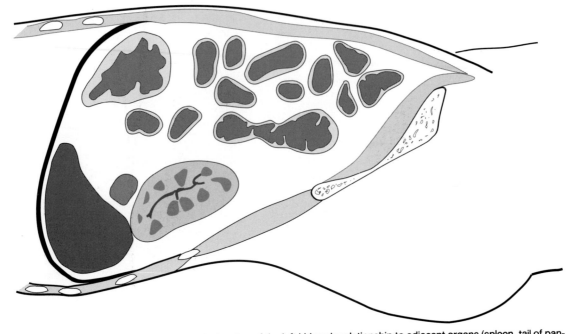

Figure 2–46. Left kidney. Demonstrates the location of the left kidney in relationship to adjacent organs (spleen, tail of pancreas, and bowel).

with suspected renal colic is to assess the presence or absence of hydronephrosis and hydroureter. Figures 2–47A–D and 2-48 illustrate the typical appearance of an acutely obstructed kidney seen in long and transverse section. The hyperreflective collecting system is seen to be distended by the homogeneous black central areas, which represent echo-free fluid within the renal pelvis. The renal pelvis only appears this way if abnormal. Figure 2–49 illustrates the appearance of a chronically obstructed kidney. The large, almost round, echo-free black areas seen in static sections might be thought to be fluid-filled cysts. Through real-time scanning at different levels within the kidney, these areas could be seen to be continuous with the collecting system. The normal ureter is not ordinarily visualized in the usual bedside scan, but the dilated ureter is sometimes seen. Figure 2–50 demonstrates this.

Although most episodes of acute colic are caused by small (2 to 4 mm) stones in the distal ureter, calcifications within the kidney itself are rather commonly found in those patients with stone disease. Although obstruction of part of the calyceal system by a proximal stone within the pelvis certainly can cause symptoms, it is relatively unlikely that intrarenal calcifications

such as those seen in Figure 2–51A–D are by themselves the cause of the acute painful episode. Such intrarenal calculi are visualized as very reflective structures, often with shadowing. In the absence of surrounding fluid, however, these are not as easy to detect as biliary calculi. Bilateral evidence of hydronephrosis is, of course, less likely to be caused by two discrete ureteral events than by bladder outlet obstruction. Figures 2–52A and B and 2–53A and B demonstrate hydronephrosis from new and long-standing obstruction. A typical finding, not usually seen with acute obstruction, is thinning of the renal medulla. It should also be recalled that hydronephrosis, sometimes of a surprising degree, can be found during normal pregnancy, especially on the right side (Fig. 2–54A and B) and with an overdistended bladder. Figures 2–55A and B and 2–56A and B show patients with isolated renal cysts and polycystic kidneys. The characteristics that distinguish cysts from hydronephrosis are described in the earlier figure legends.

A final, rather common finding that may be confused with obstruction is that of extrarenal pelvis. In this developmental variant, the collecting system lies largely outside the kidney, rather than in its usual central location sur-

Text continued on page 82

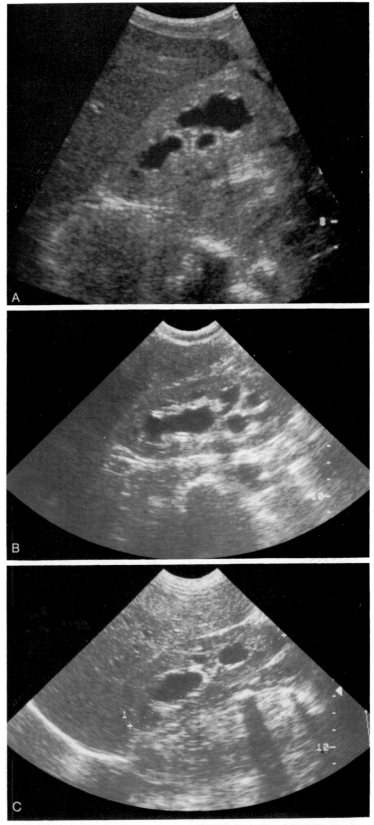

Figure 2–47. *A–D*, Acute hydronephrosis. *A–C*, These images illustrate the typical appearance of acute hydronephrosis in the longitudinal views.

Illustration continued on following page

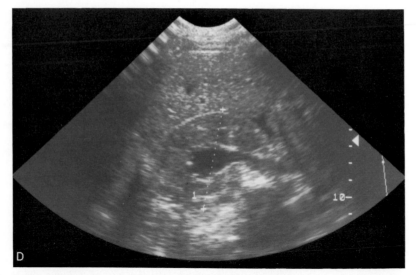

Figure 2–47 *Continued*. *D*, Transverse view. The central fluid collections in the renal pelvis are apparent; however, there is no thinning of the renal parenchyma.

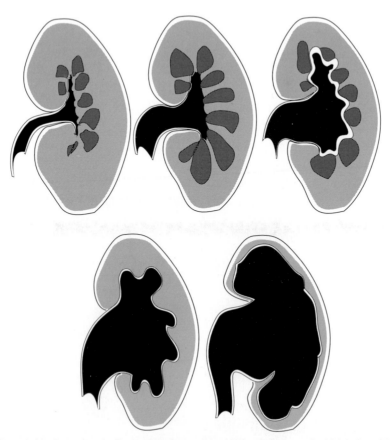

Figure 2–48. Range of hydronephrosis. Progression from minimal (*left upper*) to marked (*right lower*) hydronephrosis. With long-standing, severe hydronephrosis, there is marked dilatation of the renal pelvis and marked thinning of the remaining renal parenchyma.

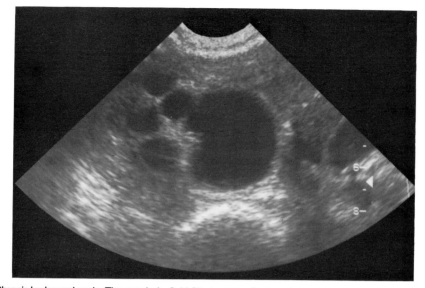

Figure 2-49. Chronic hydronephrosis. The anechoic, fluid-filled spaces displace the renal parenchyma with long-standing hydronephrosis. In contrast to the patient with polycystic kidney disease, these fluid-filled areas communicate.

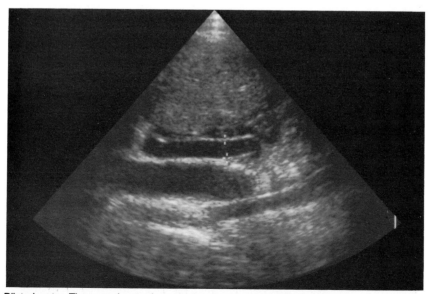

Figure 2-50. Dilated ureter. The normal ureter is rarely visualized, and the dilated ureter is only occasionally seen with ultrasound imaging. The presence of hydronephrosis is used as a marker of ureteral dilatation.

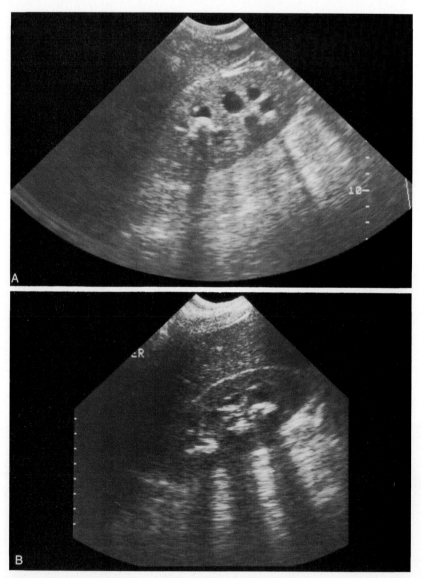

Figure 2–51. *A–D*, Intrarenal calcifications. *A* and *B*, Renal stones within the parenchyma with some evidence of hydrone-phrosis.

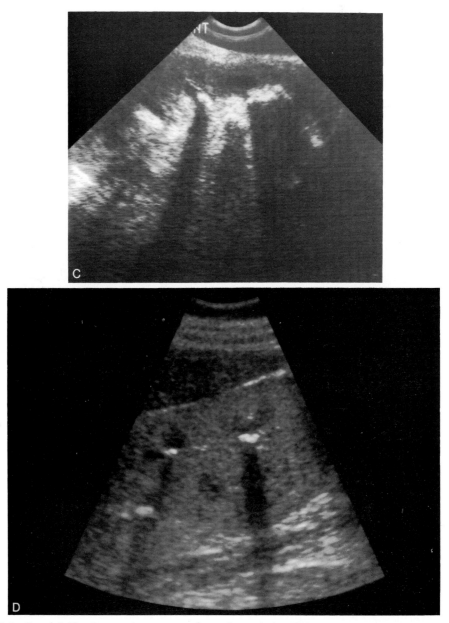

Figure 2-51 *Continued. C*, The ultrasound appearance of a staghorn calculus within a transplanted kidney. *D*, The ultrasound appearance of papillary necrosis with multiple echogenic foci located at the tips of the medullary pyramids, with posterior acoustic shadowing.

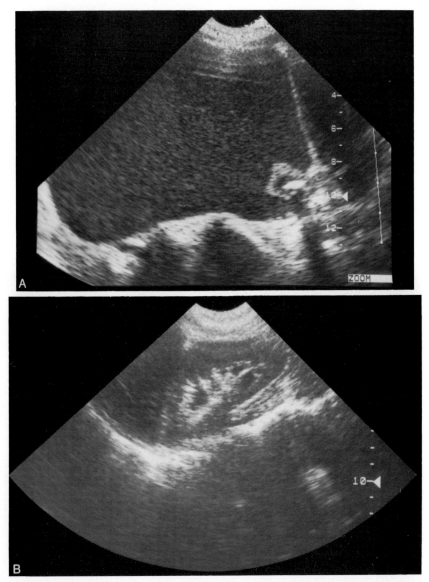

Figure 2–52. *A* and *B*, Dermoid tumor with hydronephrosis. *A*, The ultrasound appearance of a dermoid tumor. Note the echogenic foci with posterior acoustic shadowing, which represents a tooth. *B*, The consequences of ureteral obstruction on the kidney. There is mild hydronephrosis with preservation of the renal parenchyma, suggesting relatively new or partial obstruction.

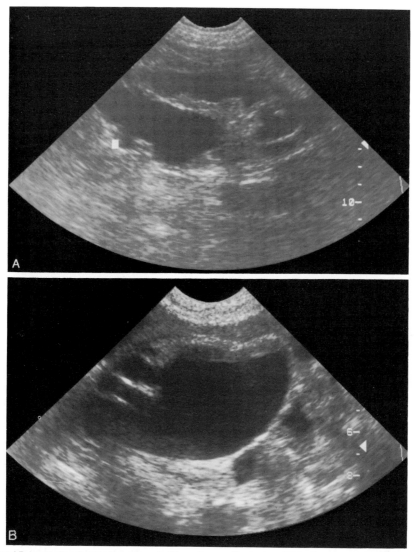

Figure 2–53. *A* and *B*, Long-standing hydronephrosis. These images illustrate striking distortion of the renal architecture with thinning of the renal parenchyma. This degree of architectural distortion is seen only with long-standing obstruction.

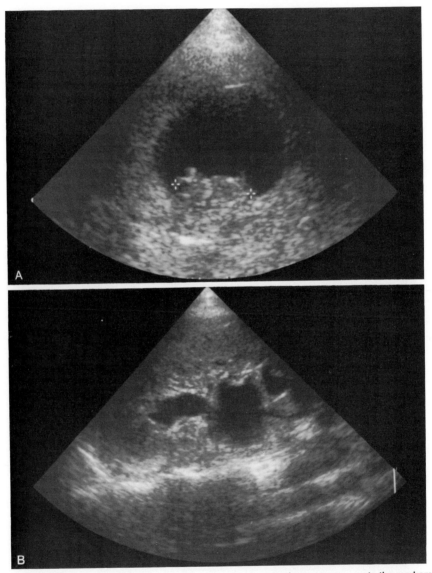

Figure 2–54. *A* and *B*, Pregnancy causing mild hydronephrosis. *A*, An intrauterine pregnancy; note the markers measuring the crown–rump length. The mechanical pressure of the uterus on the ureters is thought to cause partial obstruction. This occurs more commonly to the right kidney (90%) than the left (67%). *B*, A mild degree of hydronephrosis as a result of this pregnancy.

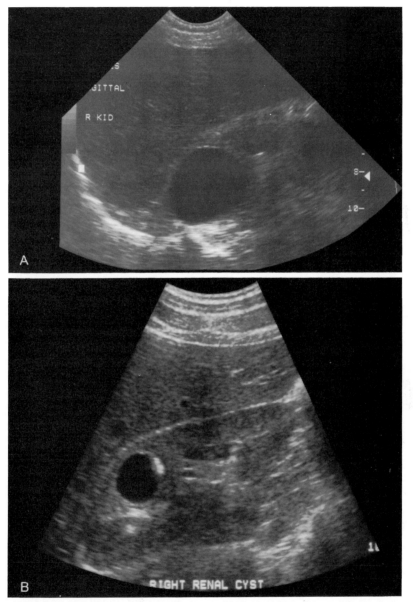

Figure 2–55. *A* and *B*, Renal cysts. These cysts arise in the renal cortex and are more commonly single rather than multiple. They are usually just incidental findings on imaging studies, but occasionally they present as a mass on physical examination.

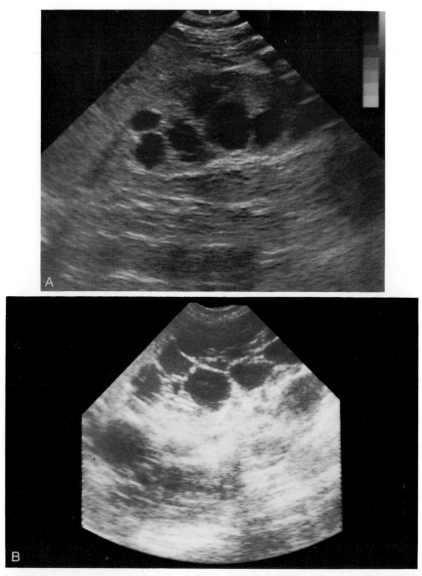

Figure 2–56. A and B, Polycystic kidneys. Adult polycystic kidney disease is inherited as an autosomal dominant trait occurring in approximately 1 of 500 individuals. These cysts enlarge with age, thereby compressing the renal parenchyma. Other complications include infection, renal stones, and cyst rupture. Liver cysts are found in one quarter to one half of these patients. Death due to polycystic kidney disease is most commonly secondary to uremia, followed by intracranial hemorrhage (aneurysms). Adult polycystic kidney disease usually becomes clinically apparent by the fourth decade of life, and ultrasound can be used to identify asymptomatic family members with this disorder.

rounded by medulla. Extrarenal pelvis may be obstructed or not obstructed, and by itself is benign. In fact, obstruction of a collecting system with an extrarenal pelvis might be expected to cause less damage and perhaps be less painful than obstruction of an intrarenal structure. Figures 2–57A and B and 2–58A and B illustrate a naturally occurring pelvic kidney and transplanted pelvic kidneys with and without hydronephrosis.

Although stones are unlikely to be visualized during bedside scanning as they pass through the ureter, there is one place where the absence of overlying bowel gas and the presence of an excellent acoustic window may allow direct documentation of the calculus. This is at the uretero-vesical junction, where the stone commonly hangs up, passing the interstitial portion of its course, within the bladder wall. Figure 2–59 illustrates a case where the stone has passed through the uretero-vesical junction into the bladder.

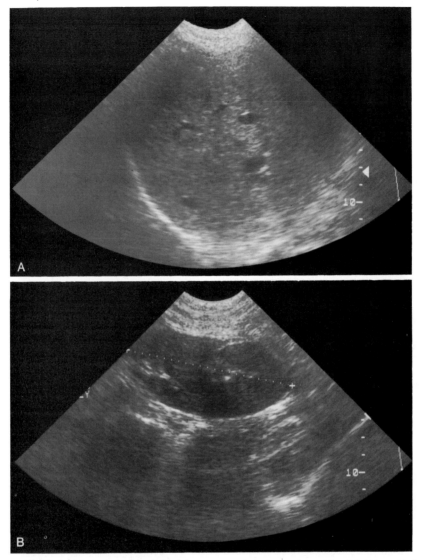

Figure 2–57. A and B, Pelvic kidney. A, A scan of the right upper quadrant in a patient with pelvic kidney. Notice the absence of renal parenchyma below the liver. B, A subsequent scan confirmed the pelvic location.

Clinical Considerations

The argument is sometimes made that there is never any indication to perform emergency ultrasound or intravenous pyelography for renal colic because (1) the acute treatment (i.e., analgesics) will be the same no matter what is found; (2) short-term renal obstruction (hours to days) does not cause irreversible kidney damage; and (3) disposition of the patient is determined by the clinical status rather than by what is recorded on x-ray film or printed from an ultrasound monitor. Although few emergency physicians (and even fewer patients with acute

renal colic!) would agree with these tenets, it is useful to critically examine such arguments in order to define how emergency ultrasound can reasonably be expected to benefit the emergency physician and his or her patient. One serious problem with the above approach is that it assumes the diagnosis is clear. In the real world of emergency medicine, this is often not the case. Furthermore, when a pain is of such intensity that acute renal colic is the prime diagnosis, any other disease process that is causing this pain is likely to be quite serious and would very well require some management other than anal-

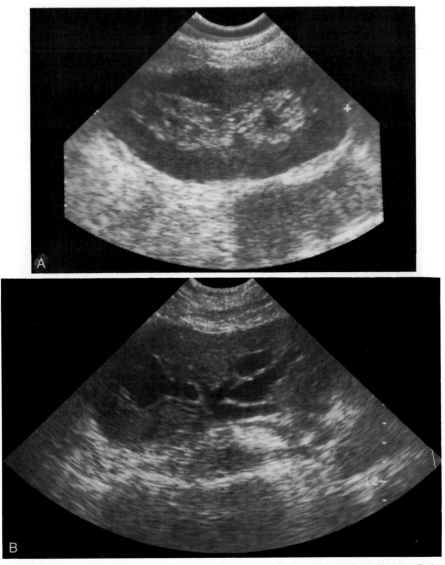

Figure 2–58. *A* and *B*, Transplanted kidneys. *A*, Ultrasound appearance of a normal transplanted kidney. *B*, A transplanted kidney with hydronephrosis.

gesics to avoid significant impairment. Dissecting aneurysms, perforated ulcers, acute embolic disease, and retroperitoneal bleeds are only a few of the common conditions that mimic acute renal colic, and each of them requires different therapy. It should be realized that, with a common condition such as renal colic, even if the certainty of diagnosis for those patients not being scanned or radiographed were 95% (and there is no reason to suspect it would be that high), this figure would still represent several thousand patients who were misdiagnosed annually with potentially serious results. One clear-cut indication for an imaging procedure is

a significant question regarding the diagnosis. It must be acknowledged that renal colic is one of the conditions most frequently faked by patients malingering for some secondary gain, either in order to be admitted or to receive narcotic analgesics. Although delaying the true diagnosis by many hours or a few days might not endanger such people, it clearly would be an extremely inappropriate utilization of resources.

In this regard, it should be emphasized exactly what normal renal ultrasound means in the patient claiming to have severe flank pain. It does not mean that the patient has no pain; it

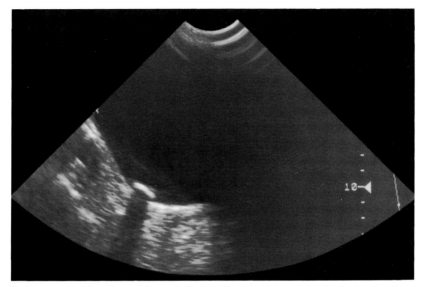

Figure 2-59. Bladder stones. There is an echogenic focus with posterior acoustic shadowing consistent with a bladder stone. These calculi are either renal stones that pass through the ureter or stones that develop primarily in the bladder. Infections, foreign bodies in the bladder, and bladder stasis predispose to the formation of primary bladder stones.

does not even mean that the patient does not have renal calculi. But, in the normally hydrated patient, absence of any evidence of dilatation virtually rules out acute renal colic as the cause of severe pain. In almost every case, this knowledge markedly changes the patient's emergency department and subsequent management. The question of hematuria is relevant here. The vast majority of patients with acute renal colic have hematuria demonstrable by dipstick or urinalysis. The 5 to 10% of patients with renal colic who do not have hematuria on initial presentation have traditionally been thought to have high-grade obstruction. Therefore, in the patient with no hematuria who complains of severe flank pain, an ultrasound examination showing no evidence of tract dilatation is inconsistent with the diagnosis of renal colic.

At least two studies have suggested the use of ultrasound as a component of a reasonable, cost-effective imaging approach. Even accepting that the diagnosis is acute renal colic, the argument that both management and patient disposition are based solely on clinical criteria is not in accord with current practice. For example, the patient in whom a large stone is noted through ultrasound or IVP is likely to be admitted promptly to the hospital with an expectation of definitive therapy by either lithotripsy or in-

vasive urologic procedure; a patient with a similar degree of distress with only a small stone (less than 3 mm) is more likely to be treated as an outpatient because there is a clear and inverse relationship between the size of the stone and the ability to pass the stone. Stones of less than 3 or 4 mm almost always pass spontaneously; larger stones may not. Also, in patients in whom ultrasound or IVP reveals an absence or a nonfunctioning contralateral kidney, the urgency to relieve the obstructing calculus is markedly greater. The issue is even more clearcut when suspicion of infection is superimposed on obstruction. In such cases, documentation of the obstruction and prompt urologic consultation are mandatory. Disposition (either inpatient or outpatient) based only on the clinical state simply is not in accord with the practice of most urologists. Current practice dictates that almost all patients, especially patients with a new diagnosis of renal colic or those admitted to a urologic service for that diagnosis, have it confirmed by an imaging procedure. It perhaps could be debated whether this should be the standard practice, but the fact is that failure to have IVP or ultrasound documentation on an emergent basis often denies the patient prompt, in-hospital care with all that implies in terms of monitoring, nursing, hydration, and analgesia.

Common Errors in Scanning the Kidney

1. Failure to scan the contralateral kidney for evidence of obstruction when hydronephrosis is noted on the symptomatic side
2. Mistaking prominent renal pyramids for hydronephrosis
3. Mistaking prominent renal pyramids for multiple small cysts
4. Interpreting an extensive extrarenal pelvis as a sign of obstruction
5. Failure to look for perinephric extravasation
6. Confusing normal renal arteries for the not normally visible ureter
7. Overdiagnosing hydronephrosis in the presence of a full bladder
8. Failure to appreciate the renal origin of a large cystic structure due to distortion of the normal anatomy
9. Failure to scan through the urinary bladder for a stone at the uretero-vesicle junction
10. Inability to visualize the left kidney completely because of transducer position anterior to the left posterior axillary line

SELECTED READINGS

Brennan R, Curtis J, Kurtz A, et al: Use of tomography and ultrasound in the diagnosis of nonopaque renal calculi. JAMA 1980;244:594.

Ellenbogen P, Talner L, Leopold G, et al: Sensitivity of ultrasound in detecting urinary tract obstruction. AJR 1978;130:731.

Erwin B, Carroll B, Sommer G: Renal colic: The role of ultrasound in initial evaluation. Radiology 1984;152:147.

Haddad MC, Sharif HS, Shahed MS, et al: Renal colic: Diagnosis and outcome. Radiology 1992;184:83–88.

Sanders RC, Conrad MR: The ultrasonic characteristics of the renal pelvicalyceal echo complex. J Clin Ultrasound 1977;5:372–377.

Sinclair D, Wilson S, Toi A, et al: The evaluation of suspected renal colic: Ultrasound scan versus excretory urography. Ann Emerg Med 1989;18:556–559.

ABDOMINAL ANEURYSMS

Emergency department patients presenting with abdominal aortic aneurysms vary from the hale and healthy 50-year-old man with an incidentally discovered abdominal mass to the critically ill octogenarian writhing in pain and barely maintaining a systolic pressure equal to his age. Emergency ultrasound examination of the aorta may be appropriate for both patients.

The aortic mass presents several distinct problems for the emergency physician, and there is no doubt that bedside ultrasound provides some solutions in situations where traditional options are not satisfactory. Without access to emergency ultrasound, the emergency physician is in the unenviable situation where the proper resources are not available quickly enough to make a decision that may very likely precipitate or prevent a fatal outcome. Ironically, improvements in surgical therapy have had the effect of restricting these highly specialized and high-risk operations to a somewhat limited number of referral centers and thus has made the problem for the emergency physician outside of a major center more acute. In such situations, when confirmation of diagnosis is required in order to transfer the patient, emergency ultrasound can play an indispensable role. With the possible exception of pericardial tamponade, there is no other condition in which the special capabilities of sonography are of such striking benefit.

Sonographic Considerations

Real-time sonography is well suited for visualization of the abdominal aorta; when aneurysmal dilatation is suspected, the diagnosis can very rapidly be made or refuted in most cases. Although traditional aortography or contrast CT gives more detailed information regarding the anatomy of the lesion, these techniques are often not immediately available or the patient may be too unstable to leave the emergency department for performance of such studies. Using a standard 3.5-MHz transducer, the abdominal aorta usually can be visualized in its entire extent to the bifurcation of the iliacs. Frequently, visualization down the iliacs is possible as well. Figure 2–60 shows the typical appearance of a normal aorta in the mid-abdominal sagittal scan. The vena cava is usually noted just to the right of the aorta (Fig. 2–61) and, in its more cephalad portion, it assumes an intrahepatic location. Distinction between the two structures can be accomplished in several ways. As indicated in Figures 2–62A and B, the aorta ordinarily is seen as a thicker-walled structure than the inferior vena cava and generally is not compressible with probe pressure. Of course, the aorta is actively pulsatile, but transmitted pulsations from both the aorta and the right

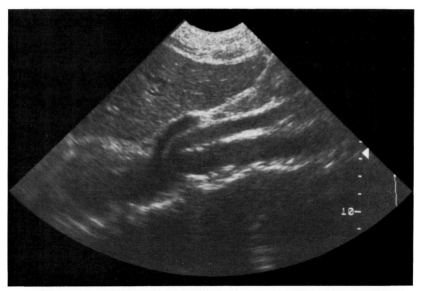

Figure 2–60. Normal abdominal aorta. Longitudinal scan of the abdominal aorta demonstrating the take-off of the celiac axis and the superior mesenteric artery. The aorta is an anechoic, tapering structure that divides at the level of the umbilicus into the iliac arteries.

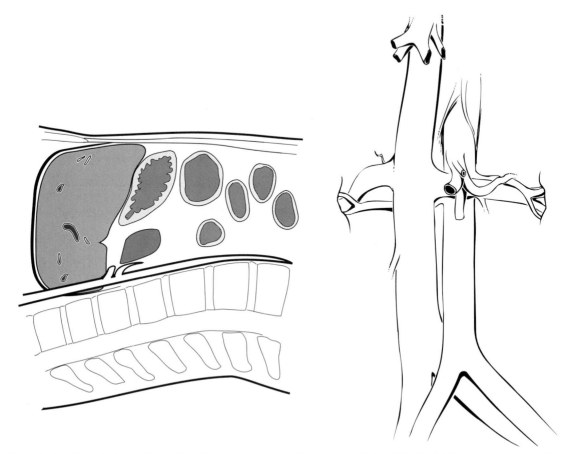

Figure 2–61. Abdominal aorta. Its relationship to adjacent organs. The vena cava is located to the right (patient's perspective) of the abdominal aorta.

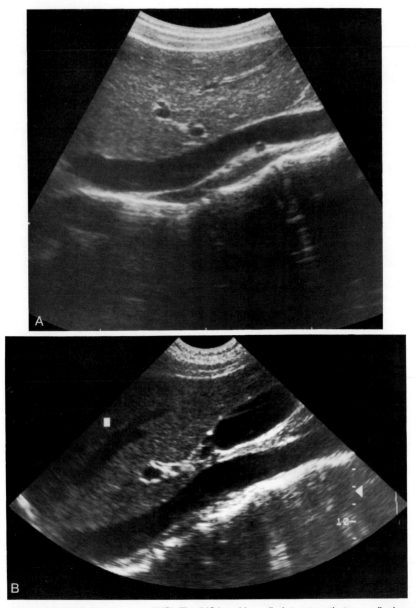

Figure 2-62. *A* and *B,* Normal inferior vena cava (IVC). The IVC is a thin-walled structure that normally decreases in size on deep inspiration. It is located on the right side of aorta and curves anteriorly as it passes through the diaphragm. *A,* Both the IVC and a small portion of the aorta (just posterior to the IVC). *B,* The intrahepatic location of the IVC as it passes cephalad. The gallbladder is anterior to the inferior vena cava in the right portion of this image.

atrium and ventricle cause pulsations of the vena cava as well, which makes this distinction less obvious than might be expected. With experience, however, the more gentle, undulating nature of the vena cava's motion can be differentiated from the more forceful, centripetal contractions of the aorta itself. The diameter of the inferior vena cava tends to be greater than that of the aorta, and the normal aorta tapers as

it progresses more distally, whereas the vena cava actually gets somewhat larger as it approaches the renal vessels. The normal aorta is no larger, and often considerably smaller, than 3 cm external diameter, even at the level of the diaphragm. At the level of the bifurcation (Fig. 2-63*A* and *B*), a diameter to 1 to 1.5 cm is common. The origins of the celiac axis, superior mesenteric artery, and renal arteries can be ap-

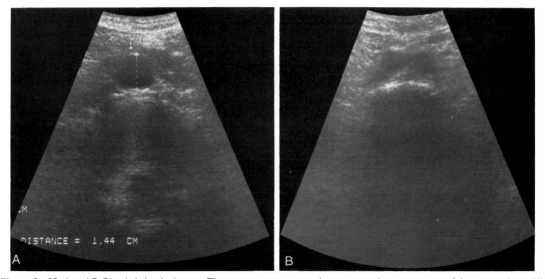

Figure 2–63. *A* and *B*, Distal abdominal aorta. These transverse scans demonstrate the appearance of the aorta prior to (*A*) and immediately after its bifurcation (*B*).

preciated in both long axis and cross section (Figs. 2–64*A* and *B* and 2–65). Loss of the normal proximal-to-distal taper (earliest sign) or a diameter greater than 3 cm indicates the presence of an abdominal aortic aneurysm. All measurements are from the outer wall. Significant aneurysms are ordinarily 5 cm or more in diameter, with a fusiform shape. True dissections sometimes occur with abdominal aneurysms and a flap can sometimes be visualized with ultrasound, but the vast majority of lesions are seen as saccular dilatations with an echo-free lumen. In many cases, thrombus is noted in the lesion, and arteriosclerotic changes in the wall are common (Figs. 2–66 and 2–67). Inhomogeneous hyperechoic shadows representing fibrin and blood components that accumulate around the weakened aortic wall can sometimes be seen, and the components of the spine are often noted incidentally immediately posterior to the aorta. The surface of the vertebral bodies, composed of highly reflective bone, appear as a bright region (Fig. 2–68), whereas the intervertebral disks, good transmitters of ultrasound, appear as just the opposite. Almost all abdominal aortic aneurysms are infrarenal, and attempts to document their location and extent as related to major vessels should be made. Figure 2–69 shows a typical abdominal aortic aneurysm with its origin 1 cm distal to the take-off of the superior mesenteric artery.

By using gentle pressure to press and displace more superficial structures, the abdominal aorta usually can be visualized in its entirety; this of course excludes the diagnosis of aortic aneurysms, but not the diagnosis of a true dissection (Fig. 2–70). In some cases, intervening bowel gas precludes a complete examination and the diagnosis cannot be excluded. The sonographer recognizes when that occurs so that there should be very few false negatives. Identification of the abdominal aortic aneurysm itself is usually unequivocal (Figs. 2–71 and 2–72). There is simply no other 5- or 6-cm pulsating structure with which it is likely to be confused. There are studies (including emergency department studies) that have confirmed the accuracy of the sonographic diagnosis of aneurysms and the ability to correctly assess the length, width and, to a lesser degree, the extent of the lesions. In one emergency department study, portable bedside sonography was performed by a radiologist on patients presenting with pain, shock, and suspicion of an abdominal mass. Within 60 seconds, all but one of 32 abdominal aortic aneurysms were correctly identified. Two thirds of these received emergency surgery. In all but one case, operative findings confirmed that it was justified.

It might be noted here that the time-honored, cross-table lateral plain radiograph of the abdomen obtained to visualize calcium in the wall of

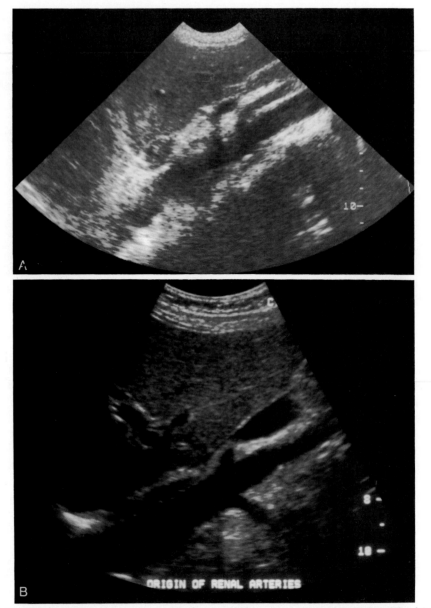

Figure 2-64. *A* and *B*, Normal longitudinal view of abdominal aorta. These images demonstrate the origin of the celiac axis, superior mesenteric artery, and renal arteries.

the aortic aneurysm plays an ever-diminishing role in modern emergency practice. When used as a test for aneurysm, studies have shown a very low sensitivity (i.e., it could never be used to rule out the diagnosis). In a setting where no other imaging techniques are available, identification of an abdominal aortic aneurysm on plain radiographs is confirmatory for the presence of an abdominal aortic aneurysm, but it is far inferior to ultrasound in its ability to confirm symptomatic abdominal aortic aneurysm.

Clinical Considerations

Emergency department patients with abdominal aortic aneurysm fall into three rather distinct groups. First, there are those who are asymptomatic; the mass is discovered incidentally either on physical or x-ray examinations. Second, there are patients who do have symptoms, either abdominal or back pain, but have no cardiovascular instability. Third, there are patients who have pain, which is usually severe, and have or have recently had signs of cardiovascu-

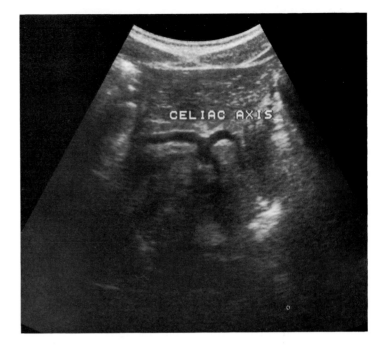

Figure 2–65. Origin of the celiac axis. This transverse scan demonstrates the ultrasound appearance of the celiac axis as it comes off of the abdominal aorta.

lar instability such as syncope, shock, or acidosis. Because the mortality rate of ruptured abdominal aortic aneurysms is essentially 100% and because the strongest predictor of mortality is the preoperative cardiovascular status of the patient, the goal of the emergency physician is quite clear: he or she must do whatever is necessary in his or her particular institution to get the patient operated on as quickly as possible. Even if the vital signs have normalized and the pain

has remitted, it is likely that deterioration, which is often catastrophic, will recur, although it is not possible to predict when. Even when the diagnosis may be obvious to the emergency physician, the reality is that confirmation of the diagnosis is often required before an operation is performed. Exceptions to this are patients who have just arrested or those who are frankly moribund on presentation to the emergency department. For the patient with stable vital signs

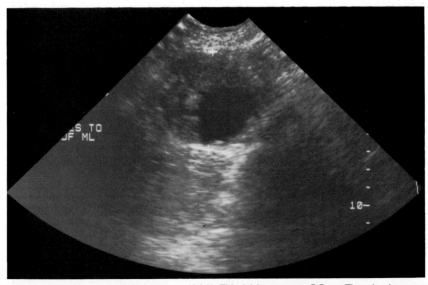

Figure 2–66. Thrombus in abdominal aortic aneurysm (AAA). This AAA measures 5.5 cm. There is a large amount of intraluminal thrombus that appears more echogenic than the small true lumen of the aorta.

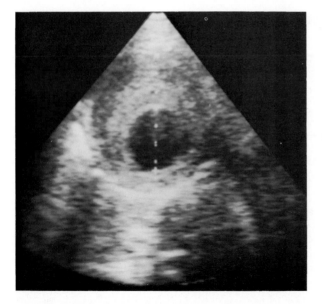

Figure 2–67. Thrombus in a rupturing aortic aneurysm (AAA). This is an image of a rupturing AAA. The internal lumen measures only 3.6 cm, because there is a large amount of intraaortic thrombus, whereas the external diameter measures 7.8 cm. Three quarters of rupturing AAA burst retroperitoneally, whereas one quarter have intraperitoneal rupture. The free intraperitoneal rupture is easy to visualize with ultrasound; however, retroperitoneal rupture (present in this case) is more difficult to identify. Bedside sonography is used in large part to identify the risk of rupture based on aneurysm size. A recent study found that 25% of abdominal aortic aneurysms measuring greater than 5 cm ruptured in the subsequent 5 years, whereas no ruptures occurred in the 130 aneurysms measuring less than 5 cm.

and who recently had cardiovascular instability, immediate bedside ultrasound in the emergency department is often the most appropriate initial step. Standard resuscitation measures can continue for the few minutes or moments it requires for the ultrasound examination and, if the diagnosis is confirmed, actions such as calling a helicopter, paging the operating room, notifying the surgeon, and preparing the cardiopulmonary bypass team can proceed immediately.

There are two potential disadvantages to this course of action. One is that the information obtained by ultrasound study is not as detailed as that obtained with aortography or CT (although no study has indicated that outcome is adversely affected). The second disadvantage is that the surgeon may insist on contrast study prior to operation. Even in this latter event, having the lesion defined by ultrasound will facilitate performance of the operation if, as so often happens, the patient suddenly deterio-

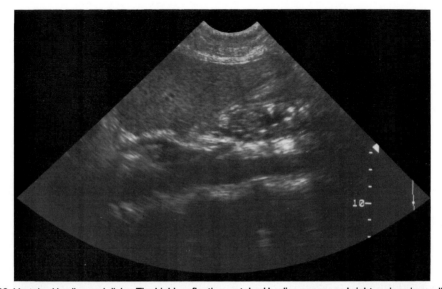

Figure 2–68. Vertebral bodies and disks. The highly reflective vertebral bodies appear as bright regions immediately posterior to the abdominal aorta, whereas the intravertebral disks are dark, because they are good transmitters of ultrasound waves.

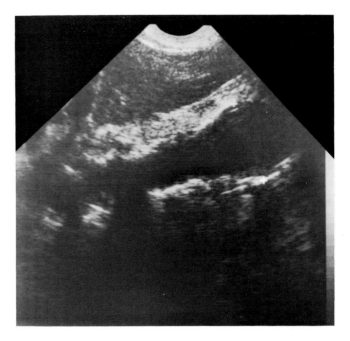

Figure 2–69. Infrarenal abdominal aortic aneurysm (AAA). Most AAAs occur in elderly men with atherosclerotic vascular disease. Greater than 95% of these occur distal to the renal arteries. This ultrasound image demonstrates a 4.7-cm fusiform AAA in the typical infrarenal location.

rates prior to completion of the contrast study. Individual circumstances justify other courses of action. For example, if bedside ultrasound is unavailable and the contrast examination entails no more delay than a formal ultrasound examination in the radiology department, it makes sense to proceed directly to the more detailed study. In most cases, however, documentation by immediate ultrasound saves time and provides a margin of safety, even if a second imaging procedure is decided on prior to operation.

For patients in the second category—those with only mild abdominal symptoms—there are often questions regarding the diagnosis. In such instances, ultrasound not only rules out abdominal aortic aneurysm, but it may be helpful in establishing a second diagnosis such as renal colic or retroperitoneal hematoma, which may mimic an aneurysm. Also, documentation of the location and size of the aneurysm may aid in dictating the urgency for repair in this group. Opinions vary somewhat, but there is general agreement that large aneurysms, more than 6 cm and definitely more than 7 cm, are at much greater risk (up to 76% in one series) for early rupture than are smaller lesions. For the third group of patients, those with an abdominal mass but no symptoms, ultrasound obtained during the emergency department visit is useful in directing appropriate follow-up. The physician must ascertain if the patient is in fact asymptomatic and has not failed to mention, for example, the recent onset of back pain. The presence of symptoms is the strongest predictor of risk for early rupture.

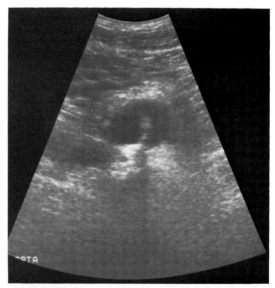

Figure 2–70. Abdominal aortic dissection. This image demonstrates a small flap in the abdominal aorta that represents an aortic dissection. This is almost always an extension of thoracic aortic disease into the abdomen. Transesophageal echocardiography and aortography are the diagnostic tests of choice for this disorder.

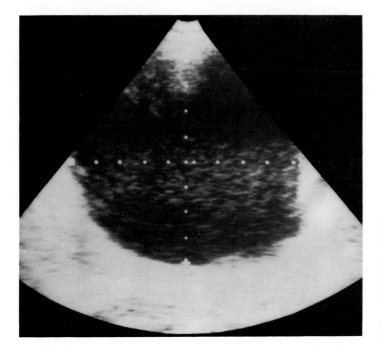

Figure 2–71. Rupturing abdominal aortic aneurysm (AAA). This is an 8.0 × 9.4 cm aneurysm that was rupturing on the patient's presentation to the emergency department. Diagnosis required no additional (other than bedside sonography) confirmatory tests prior to the patient being taken to the operating room. The ultrasound diagnosis of the AAA is reported to have a 98% accuracy.

A few other clinical points bear mentioning. For unstable patients, the standard principles of resuscitation apply, but there is controversy regarding both aggressive fluid therapy and use of the military anti-shock trousers (MAST) suit on patients hypotensive from leaking aneurysms. Concern that normalization of low but tolerable blood pressure may exacerbate rupture of the weakened aortic wall may temper enthusiasm for massive fluid replacement and vasoconstricting modalities such as a MAST suit and alpha-adrenergic agents. It should also be recalled that some patients presenting with symptoms of abdominal aortic aneurysm have, in fact, suffered thoracic aortic dissection that has extended below the diaphragm. Initial assessment of upper extremity pulses as well as lower extremity pulses and consideration of

Figure 2–72. Rupturing abdominal aortic aneurysm (AAA). This 9-cm aortic aneurysm was diagnosed by physical examination and bedside sonography. Following emergency department stabilization, the patient was transported directly to the operating room for emergency surgery.

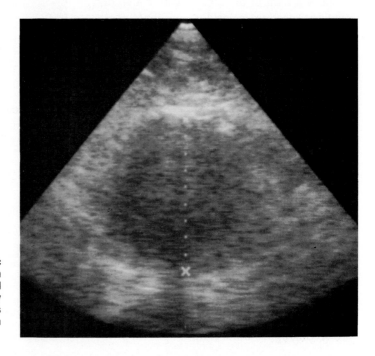

transesophageal echocardiography are in order (see Chapter 3, "Other Cardiac Applications").

A recent radiology text introduces the chapter on abdominal aortic aneurysm in this way: "Urgent real-time sonography is the imaging method of choice in evaluating patients with abdominal pain, hypotension, and suspected rupture of an abdominal aortic aneurysm. Ideally, sonographic consideration is performed rapidly with portable equipment in the emergency room at the time of initial evaluation and resuscitation." Clearly, bedside emergency department ultrasound for the aneurysm patient is not just state of the art: it may become a standard of care.

Common Errors in Scanning for Abdominal Aortic Aneurysm

1. Failure to adequately compress overlying bowel with probe pressure
2. Confusion of the vena cava with the aorta due to transmitted pulsations
3. Overestimating the aneurysmal width due to lack of a true cross section
4. Misinterpreting acoustic enhancement distal to the aorta as evidence of leakage
5. Failure to move the transducer off the sagittal plane while following a tortuous aorta
6. Neglecting to note the take-off of the renal arteries
7. Not measuring external diameter (outer wall to outer wall)
8. Reluctance to move the transducer far laterally in an attempt to visualize an aorta that is obscured by overlying bowel gas
9. Neglecting to visualize the bifurcation of the iliacs
10. Confusing artifact for thrombus

SELECTED READINGS

Abdominal Aortic Aneurysm

Conrad M, David G, Green C, et al: Real-time ultrasound in the diagnosis of acute dissecting aneurysm of the abdominal aorta. AJR 1979;132:115.
Jeffrey R: CT and Sonography of the Acute Abdomen. New York: Raven Press, 1989.
Laroy L, Cormia P, Mattalon T, et al: Imaging of abdominal aortic aneurysms. AJR 1989;152:785–792.
Pearce WH, Yao IS: Noninvasive diagnosis of vascular diseases. Surg Clin North Am 1990;70:1.
Schlager D, Lazzaresch G, Whitten D, et al: A prospective study of ultrasonography in the ED by emergency physicians. Am J Emerg Med 1994;12:185–189.
Shuman WP, Hastrup W Jr, Kohler TR, et al: Suspected leaking abdominal aortic aneurysm: Use of sonography in the emergency room. Radiology 1988;168:117–119.
Vouden P, Wilinson D, Ausobsky J, Kester R: A comparison of three imaging techniques in the assessment of an abdominal aortic aneurysm. J Cardiovasc Surg 1989; 30:891–896.

HEMOPERITONEUM

Although ultrasound was first used to detect hemoperitoneum in blunt abdominal trauma almost 25 years ago, it is only in the last 5 years that this technique has been widely accepted. In the United States especially, recognition of intraabdominal blood has been accomplished almost exclusively by diagnostic peritoneal lavage (DPL) and CT. This is changing rapidly because many investigations both here and abroad have clearly documented that emergency department ultrasound can be at least as sensitive as DPL, performed much more rapidly, and allows for a noninvasive diagnosis even in the unstable patient. Diagnosis of hemoperitoneum may be considered the newest of the primary emergency department applications, but it is also one of the best studied; almost two dozen prospective, controlled series have been reported. Now that the potential of ultrasound in blunt abdominal trauma has been established (it has virtually replaced DPL in many European trauma centers), research attention is being directed toward more specific questions such as defining the optimal scanning technique, quantifying the learning curve, and identifying particular organ injury.

General Considerations

It has long been established that clinical examination, standard radiographs, and routine blood tests are incapable of accurately identifying which patients with blunt abdominal trauma require surgical intervention. Both DPL and CT are highly accurate in making this determination; however, each has serious limitations. For CT, issues of expense, availability, expertise in interpretation, and unsuitability for the unstable patient have continued to be major problems, particularly outside of trauma centers. DPL obviates some of these concerns, but most objective observers agree that both the time required to obtain interpretable results and the incidence of procedure-related complications are significant.

The development of high-quality, portable ultrasound units and the increasing availability of ultrasound-capable personnel (particularly in Europe and Japan, where training and use of ultrasound by general surgeons is common) are profoundly altering the traditional approach to the blunt trauma patient. Immediate ultrasound scanning is performed in the trauma bay coincident with the usual resuscitation procedures. If no intraperitoneal fluid is seen (using the criteria discussed below), the interpretation is the same as a negative DPL, with all that implies in terms of admission, transfer, and surgery. Similarly, unequivocal identification of fluid (which is assumed to represent fresh hemorrhage) is equivalent to a positive DPL. Although the gold standard in different studies has been variable, sensitivity and specificity have routinely been between 90 and 100%, with most recent reports emphasizing near-perfect specificity and somewhat lower sensitivity. As with DPL, false positives occur in the sense that no operative repair may be necessary even though hemoperitoneum is present. Also, bowel rupture results in fluid in the abdomen, which is not a true hemoperitoneum (although an operation is required). These, too, are sometimes termed false positives. Finally, differences in technique and experience are both quite relevant. Scanning has been performed using as few as one and as many as five different acoustic windows; the operators have included emergency medicine, surgery, and radiology residents, as well as attending physicians of various stripes. Data on the effect of these variables are accumulating more rapidly than for any other emergency department ultrasound application.

Sonographic Considerations

Fresh, unclotted blood appears anechoic on ultrasound; it is this black "stripe" in an abdominal location that makes the ultrasound diagnosis of hemoperitoneum. Fluids collect preferentially in a few locations within the abdominal cavity (although blood may not be as freely mobile as ascites), and these are the chief areas of concern. Figure 2–73 illustrates the patterns of free fluid movement within the abdominal cavity.

The most important and the easiest region to visualize is Morison's pouch, the potential space between the liver and the kidney (Fig. 2–74A and B). Figure 2-74C and D show typical collections of blood, seen in this region as an anechoic stripe sandwiched between the more hyperechoic Gerota's fascia and Glisson's capsule. Figure 2–75 illustrates fluid in Morison's pouch with the transducer's almost sagittal position just above the right costal margin. It might be expected that some degree of Trendelenburg positioning would maximize the amount of blood collected here, making the examination more sensitive. Figure 2–74D shows this region with a more dramatic degree of fluid.

A second region where fluid may be seen is in the left upper quadrant, also scanned longitudinally. Fluid may collect in the paracolic gutter, surrounding the left kidney, or be layered between the spleen and the kidney, as shown in Figure 2–76. It seems almost certain that scanning in more than one location increases the sensitivity appreciably. Although Morison's pouch is usually the most sensitive area for detecting fluid, the location of the trauma, subtle differences in patient positioning, prior abdominal surgery, and other unknown factors may negate this advantage in any given case.

The third common region in which to look for hemoperitoneum is over the pelvis in the region of the cul-de-sac. Because this is the most dependent portion of the supine patient (using

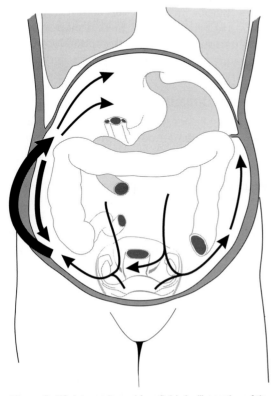

Figure 2–73. Intraperitoneal free fluid. An illustration of the pattern of free fluid movement within the abdominal cavity.

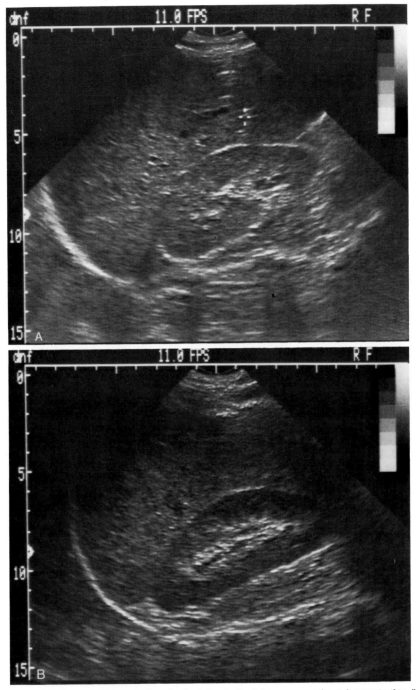

Figure 2–74. *A* and *B*, Negative studies. Normal longitudinal view in the right upper quadrant demonstrating diaphragm, liver, and kidney (left to right). No anechoic (black) stripe is visualized above the outer white border of the kidney. (From Jehle D, Guarino J, Karamanoukian H: Emergency department ultrasound in the evaluation of blunt abdominal trauma. Am J Emerg Med 1993;11:342–346.)

Illustration continued on following page

reverse Trendelenburg may be even better), this might in theory be the best location of all. Unfortunately, visualization is less than optimal unless the bladder is full. Any degree of Trendelenburg positioning is detrimental to imaging

this region as well. Figure 2–77 shows the appearance of fluid in the cul-de-sac by transabdominal scanning. In females, transvaginal ultrasound is exquisitely sensitive for visualizing fluid (less than 5 mL) in this region and does not

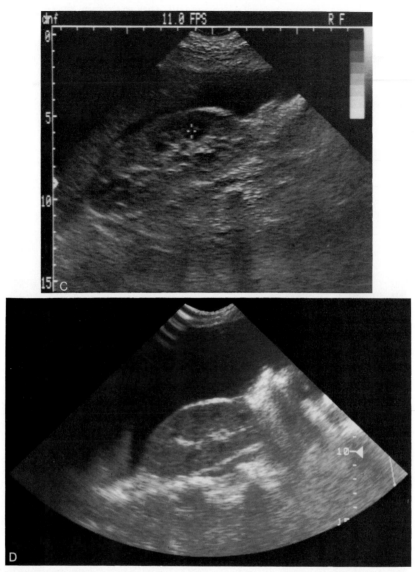

Figure 2-74 *Continued*. *C*, Positive study. Longitudinal view in right upper quadrant with anechoic stripe between the liver and the right kidney in Morison's pouch, representing intraperitoneal fluid. *D*, Large amount of fluid. This demonstrates the appearance of very large quantities of fluid in Morison's pouch.

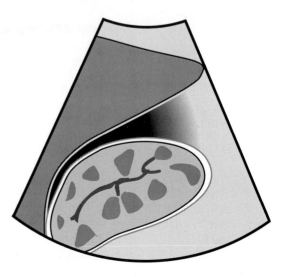

Figure 2-75. Fluid in Morison's pouch. The typical appearance of fluid in Morison's pouch as an anechoic stripe between the liver and the right kidney.

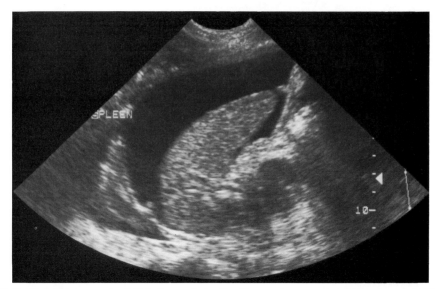

Figure 2–76. Fluid in left upper quadrant. This demonstrates the ultrasound appearance of a large amount of fluid surrounding the spleen.

require a full bladder. In males, it might be expected that transrectal ultrasound would provide a similarly sensitive view. Neither technique has been well described in the trauma setting; however, several examples of cul-de-sac fluid scanned by transvaginal ultrasound may be seen later in this chapter in the "Pelvic Applications" section.

Quantitating Hemoperitoneum

It has been surprisingly difficult to get consistent information on how much fluid is required before ultrasound visualization. Clearly, this is one way of determining how sensitive the study is. As little as 10 mL has been seen by the transabdominal route, but it appears that transabdominal ultrasound can ordinarily detect about 150 to 200 mL of free-flowing fluid. Given the time, space, and equipment constraints of a trauma resuscitation and the variable viscosity of partially defibrinated blood, the threshold for reliably diagnosing hemoperitoneum may be approximately 250 mL. In fact, it has been reported that a very thin anechoic stripe under the

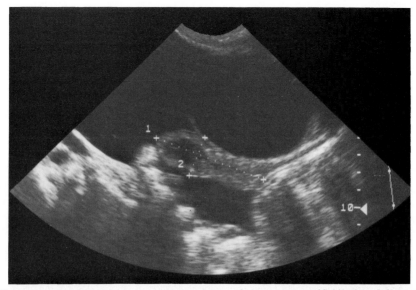

Figure 2–77. Fluid in the pelvis. This demonstrates the appearance of a large amount of fluid in the cul-de-sac posterior to the uterus on a transabdominal scan. The markers outline the dimensions of the uterus.

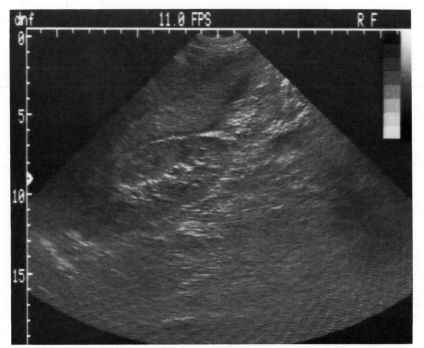

Figure 2-78. Positive study. There is a small anechoic stripe visualized in Morison's pouch representing 250 to 500 mL of free intraperitoneal blood. (From Jehle D, Guarino J, Karamanoukian H: Emergency department ultrasound in the evaluation of blunt abdominal trauma. Am J Emerg Med 1993;11:342–346.)

liver (Fig. 2–78) represents 250 mL of blood and that a stripe 0.5 cm in width (Fig. 2–79) correlates with more than 500 mL. With large amounts of blood (in the range of 1 L), the fluid is visible from almost anywhere in the abdomen. The characteristic appearance of bowel loops floating on mesentery is indicated in Figure 2–80; many organs take on an unusual appearance when they are separated and outlined by large quantities of fluid.

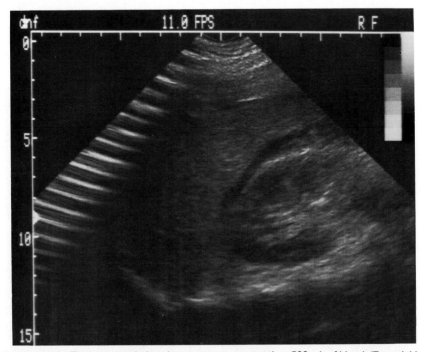

Figure 2-79. Positive study. The large anechoic stripe represents greater than 500 mL of blood. (From Jehle D, Guarino J, Karamanoukian H: Emergency department ultrasound in the evaluation of blunt abdominal trauma. Am J Emerg Med 1993;11:342–346.)

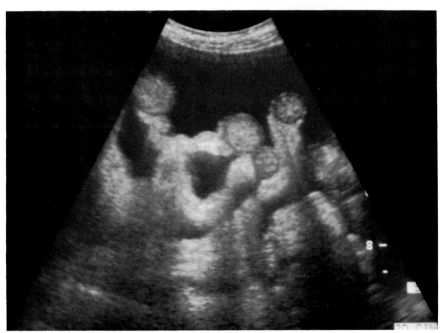

Figure 2–80. Bowel loops. These loops will float or sink in the surrounding fluid, depending on the fat and gas content of the mesentery/bowel. In the ultrasound image, the bowel is anchored posteriorly by the mesentery with fluid between the folds.

Qualitative Fluid Characteristics

Fresh blood appears anechoic. When it is free in the peritoneum (or pleural space), it has somewhat characteristic sharp angles, unlike intravascular blood (Figure 2–81). At times, blood appears to layer along an organ's surface, presumably through capillary attraction. As soon as the clotting process begins, blood begins to lose its anechoic appearance and takes on variable echoes, becoming more echoic as fibrin and degenerating cells make up a greater part of its substance (Fig. 2–82).

It is not uncommon that the presumed hemoperitoneum has regions that look noticeably echoic. In such a case, the appearance may represent (1) blood that has already started to defi-

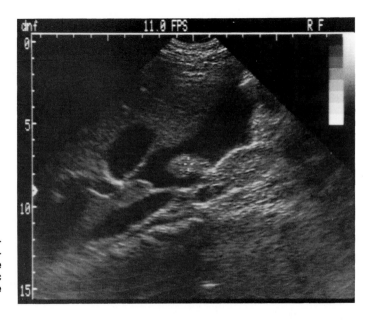

Figure 2–81. Intraperitoneal blood. This ultrasound scan demonstrates the appearance of free intraperitoneal blood in the center of the image. Note the characteristic sharp angles of the blood in contrast to the appearance of intravascular blood.

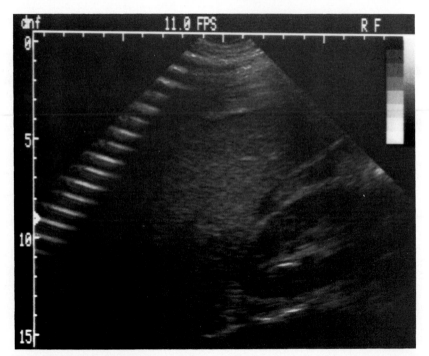

Figure 2–82. Clotting blood. The echogenic areas within the anechoic stripe illustrate the appearance of blood with small clots. (From Jehle D, Guarino J, Karamanoukian H: Emergency department ultrasound in the evaluation of blunt abdominal trauma. Am J Emerg Med 1993;11:342–346.)

brinate; (2) some fluid that is not blood, such as intestinal contents; or (3) some combination of the two. One clear advantage of using ultrasound in blunt trauma is the ability to do serial examinations. Both the quantity and quality of the blood can be seen to change with surprising rapidity. Figure 2–83 shows a trauma case that was misinterpreted as a hemoperitoneum. In retrospect, the anechoic stripe represented ascites in a patient with liver disease.

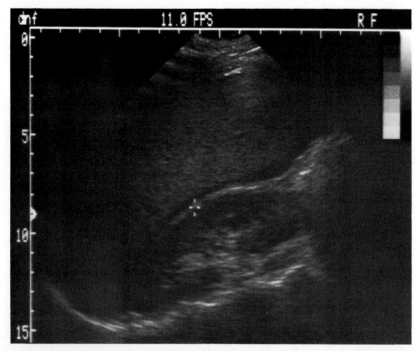

Figure 2–83. False-positive study. Anechoic stripe in Morison's pouch "misinterpreted" as intraperitoneal blood. This fluid proved to be ascitic fluid. (From Jehle D, Guarino J, Karamanoukian H: Emergency department ultrasound in the evaluation of blunt abdominal trauma. Am J Emerg Med 1993;11:342–346.)

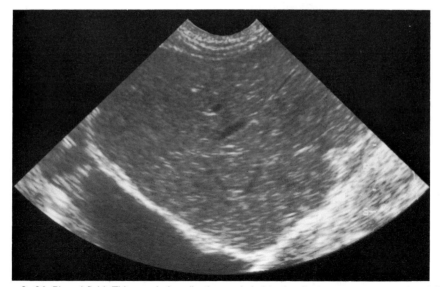

Figure 2–84. Pleural fluid. This anechoic collection cephalad to the diaphragm represents pleural fluid.

The ultrasound examination itself is usually performed with a 3.5-MHz transducer, while resuscitative efforts proceed as usual. The right upper quadrant is examined first (unless the bladder is about to be emptied, in which case the pelvis is visualized first), with the transducer either just subcostally or in an intercostal position. If no hemoperitoneum is visualized, it is quite appropriate to attempt some Trendelenburg positioning. Occasionally, fluid is seen above the diaphragm (Fig. 2–84), suggesting the diagnosis of hemothorax. At other times,

fluid may be found in a subdiaphragmatic location, rather than free in the peritoneum (Fig. 2–85). Moving on to the left side, the interface between kidney and spleen is visualized, as is the left pericolic gutter. Pelvic ultrasound, if feasible, may be performed last.

All authors agree that the entire examination is very rapid. The single-view examination takes between 30 seconds and 1 minute; even with multiple views and multiple studies, total time is less than 5 minutes. Some authors have advocated conservative management of very

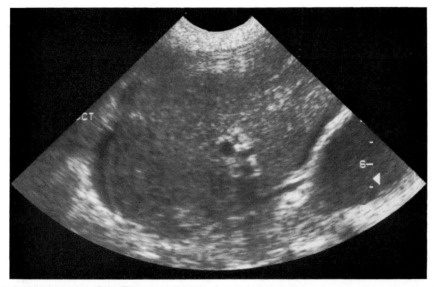

Figure 2–85. Subdiaphragmatic fluid. This anechoic stripe between the diaphragm and the liver represents subdiaphragmatic fluid. In addition, there is an anechoic stripe to the right of the liver, representing infrahepatic fluid.

small quantity hemoperitoneum with serial ultrasound (and often CT) examinations. An increasing hemoperitoneum is an indication for surgery.

Other Organ Trauma

Although ultrasound can sometimes identify the cause of the hemoperitoneum (e.g., splenic laceration, fractured kidney, liver laceration, etc.), such diagnoses are difficult even in ideal circumstances. Sensitivity for common solid organ injuries is only about 30%, and it is quite clear that CT is by far the preferred study for defining individual organ injury. Specific comments regarding the ultrasound appearance of traumatic abdominal injuries are noted in more detail in Chapter 3.

Common Errors in Scanning for Hemoperitoneum

1. Failure to scan the paracolic region as well as Morison's pouch
2. Failure to scan the pelvis if more cephalad areas are negative
3. Failure to scan from the anterior intercostal approach as well as the posterolateral
4. Failure to note echogenicity within the stripe
5. Failure to consider urine and intestinal contents as possible intraperitoneal fluids
6. Failure to consider the possibility of preexisting ascites
7. Failure to perform serial scans when initial scan is negative
8. Failure to appreciate the relative insensitivity of ultrasound for organ injury
9. Confusion of hypoechoic perinephric fat with fluid in Morison's pouch

SELECTED READINGS

Glaser K, Tschmelitsch J, Klinger P, et al: Ultrasonography in the management of blunt abdominal and thoracic trauma. Arch Surg 1994;129:743–747.

Gruessner R, Menteges B, Duber C, et al: Sonography versus peritoneal lavage in blunt abdominal trauma. J Trauma 1980;29:242–244.

Hoffmann R, Nerlich M, Muggia-Sullam M, et al: Blunt abdominal trauma in cases of multiple trauma evaluated by ultrasonography: A prospective analysis of 291 patients. J Trauma 1991;32:452–458.

Jehle D, Guarino J, Karamanoukian H: Emergency department ultrasound in the evaluation of blunt abdominal trauma. Am J Emerg Med 1993;1:342–346.

Kimura A, Otsuka T: Emergency center ultrasonography in the evaluation of hemoperitoneum: A prospective study. J Trauma 1991,31:20–23.

Rozycki GS: Prospective evaluation of surgeons' use of ultrasound in the evaluation of trauma patients. J Trauma 1993;34:516–527.

Tso P, Rodriguez A, Cooper C, et al: Sonography in blunt abdominal trauma: A preliminary progress report. J Trauma 1992;33:39–44.

Texts

With the exception of hemoperitoneum, standard ultrasound texts are the best sources for the emergency department physician seeking more detailed descriptions and additional ultrasound images relating to the primary abdominal indications. All written by radiologists (or sonographers), they vary considerably in their attempts at clinical correlation and applicability to emergency medicine.

Fleisher AC, James AE: Diagnostic Sonography: Principles and Clinical Applications. Philadelphia: W. B. Saunders, 1989. *Covers all of ultrasound, resulting in very brief but pointed and practical sections on primary abdominal indications. Well-chosen images, all with accompanying graphic and orientation icons. References superbly grouped according to specific topics.*

Goldberg B: Textbook of Abdominal Ultrasound. Baltimore: Williams & Wilkins, 1993. *Concise descriptions with many very good images. Emphasis on ultrasound appearance rather than clinical correlation and technique.*

Hagen-Ansert SL: Textbook of Diagnostic Ultrasonography, 3rd ed. St. Louis: C.V. Mosby, 1989. *Edited by a sonographer, rather than a radiologist; especially strong in technique, rather than clinical application.*

Higashi Y, Mizushima A, Matsumoto H: Introduction to Abdominal Ultrasonography. New York: Springer-Verlag, 1991. *A user-friendly soft-cover handbook that is the closest thing to a "Dubins" of ultrasound yet published. Not a reference work in any sense, it uses simple descriptions and line drawings that are very attractive to beginners in abdominal ultrasound.*

Mittelstaedt CA: Abdominal Ultrasound. New York: Churchill Livingstone, 1992. *New edition of a classic. Fine images and exceptionally detailed descriptions of ultrasound findings, often presenting quantitative data from multiple references.*

Pelvic Applications

Mark Deutchman, MD

ABNORMAL FIRST TRIMESTER PREGNANCY

There is no condition in which emergency ultrasound has found greater acceptance than in the evaluation of suspected abnormal early pregnancy. Partially — but only partially — this is due to the fact that during the first trimester of pregnancy, pain in the abdomen or pelvis with or without vaginal bleeding is such a common emergency department presentation. Many such patients do not know that they are pregnant. The emergency physician must therefore keep the diagnosis of early pregnancy and its complications in the differential diagnosis of any female patient of reproductive age. In addition to the conditions that are discussed in this chapter, virtually every other traumatic, infectious, and inflammatory condition that exists in the nongravid patient can coexist with pregnancy, sometimes obscuring both the clinical and sonographic appearance.

The most critical common diagnosis that the emergency physician must consider is that of ectopic pregnancy; much of this section is devoted to the manner in which emergency sonography may be integrated into the clinical and laboratory examination. Emergent ultrasonography dramatically increases the number of cases that can be definitively diagnosed in the emergency department and provides alternative diagnoses in many other cases. However, even with the immediate availability of diagnostic ultrasound, serum hormone testing, and specialty consultation, it may be impossible to either confirm or refute the diagnosis of an ectopic pregnancy in certain cases. In almost every case, however, the intelligent application of these tools reveals whether the patient is at low or high risk for an ectopic pregnancy and guides further inpatient or outpatient work-up.

Although the incidence of ectopic pregnancy varies strikingly in different populations, there is no question that the overall incidence is increasing. In 1970, 0.25% of all pregnancies were ectopic, quadrupling to 1% by 1985. The national epidemic of pelvic inflammatory disease is thought to play a major role, but other factors, such as current or previous intrauterine device (IUD) use, hormonal therapy, the use of fertility drugs, and previous tubal surgical procedures, have all been postulated to play a role. Even with heightened awareness of ectopic pregnancy by the medical profession and the lay public, ectopic pregnancy remains a significant cause of maternal mortality and is a major medical/legal concern, having been reported to represent the second leading cause (in dollar amounts) of awards against emergency physicians. Conversely, the timely diagnosis of ectopic pregnancy not only reduces liability, but also provides the best opportunity for the patient to receive fertility-preserving therapy.

The availability of emergency department ultrasound offers several unique advantages applicable to the subject of this and subsequent sections. First and most importantly, emergency department ultrasound can make immediate and definitive diagnoses in a large percentage of patients in whom an abnormal or complicated early pregnancy is suspected. These diagnoses include normal intrauterine pregnancy, living ectopic pregnancy, intrauterine embryonic demise, and trophoblastic disease. The use of ultrasound for these patients can greatly shorten the emergency department stay and may obviate the need for other tests and procedures such as cultures, serum human chorionic gonadotropin (hCG) levels, progesterone levels, and culdocentesis. The result can be economic savings as well as more rapid diagnosis. Second, even in cases in which the sonographic study does not provide a definitive diagnosis, ancillary findings may indicate that the patient is at high risk for ectopic pregnancy and therefore requires aggressive diagnostic measures and urgent subspecialty evaluation. Third, diagnostic ultrasound, when used by the clinician, becomes an extension of the physical examination. Not only can abnormalities detected on physical examination be clarified immediately, but the physician's pelvic examination skills can improve as a result of this repeated and immediate feedback. Use of pelvic ultrasound in this way to aid in the education of medical students and house officers is just beginning. Finally, diagnostic ultrasound can be used in early pregnancy to guide clinical procedures, including instrumentation of the uterus and culdocentesis, making them faster, more accurate, and less painful.

Terminology of Early Pregnancy

All physicians involved in the care of patients in the first trimester of pregnancy should understand the terminology used in this setting. Emergency physicians are frequently communicating with colleagues regarding therapy and disposition of their patients; therefore, both groups should use similar terms.

Pregnancy Dating. Clinicians traditionally use menstrual dating (counted from the first day of the last menstrual period); embryology books use postconception dating (counting from the day that the sperm and ovum unite, known only in cases of in vitro fertilization). A patient may use all kinds of dating, including day of intercourse, the day she first "felt" pregnant and, commonly, the date her period ended. It is therefore critical that the physician ask the patient about the first day of her last menstrual period, describing precisely what that means, because any misunderstanding can easily cause inaccuracies of more than 1 week, which may be critical in evaluating sonographic findings.

Spontaneous Abortion and Miscarriage. Spontaneous abortion and miscarriage are synonymous terms in early pregnancy and refer to spontaneous (not induced) passage of the products of conception through the cervical os.

Threatened Abortion. A threatened abortion is a pregnancy prior to 20 weeks accompanied by cramping and bleeding. Approximately half of all women with a diagnosed pregnancy have some type of bleeding, and about half of these will miscarry.

Incomplete Abortion. An incomplete abortion is that condition in which some products of conception remain within the uterus after miscarriage.

Complete Abortion. A complete abortion is that condition in which all products of conception are passed through the cervix and none remain within the uterus.

Inevitable Abortion. Inevitable abortion is a condition in which the patient's cervix is dilated (the precise amount of dilatation required varies) and products of conception are often seen exiting the cervical os.

Missed Abortion. Missed abortion is that condition in which the fetus has died and all products of conception, including placenta, membranes, and amniotic fluid, remain within the uterus.

Blighted Ovum. Blighted ovum is a frequently used but ambiguous term that formerly indicated that no embryo ever developed. A synonymous term was anembryonic pregnancy. Recent high-resolution scanning has shown that the very early embryo usually does develop and subsequently degenerates. *Embryonic resorption* is a more modern and appropriate term.

Embryonic Demise. Embryonic demise is an early pregnancy in which no fetal heart beat or motion is seen in a clearly visible embryo (dead embryo).

Trophoblastic Disease. Trophoblastic disease is a condition in which tissue of placental origin undergoes potentially malignant degeneration.

Viable. Viable properly refers to a fetus "capable of living outside the uterus" and therefore should be limited to pregnancies reaching the third or late second trimesters. First trimester pregnancies that appear normal are often loosely referred to as viable, but are more appropriately labeled as living.

Sonographic Considerations

The pregnant uterus is an ideal organ for sonographic examination. The embryo is surrounded by amniotic fluid, which provides an excellent acoustic window. Air-filled maternal structures, such as the bowel, may interfere with the ultrasound examination. They either can be pushed out of the way by a full maternal urinary bladder or avoided completely by scanning transvaginally. Transvaginal scanning has revolutionized first trimester sonography by placing the transducer closer to the object of interest and allowing the use of higher frequency transducers, which produce a more detailed image. The greater image detail available with transvaginal sonography has led to the term *sonoembryology*, reflecting the fact that what is visible sonographically reflects accurately embryologic development. Transvaginal scanning offers the added benefit of obviating the need for a full maternal urinary bladder, which is often difficult or time consuming to achieve in the emergency department. Nonetheless, it is important to keep in mind that the transvaginal approach with a high-frequency transducer is associated with a limited field of view and that some abnormalities (particularly those higher in the pelvis) are visualized better —and perhaps exclusively—by transabdominal scanning.

The choice of initial scan route, transabdominal or transvaginal, must be made on an individual basis, depending on local practices, the skill of the examiner, and the clinical condition of the patient. Both types of scanning may yield a definitive diagnosis if used first. Transvaginal scanning is more sensitive in detecting small amounts of cul-de-sac fluid, in defining early intrauterine pregnancies, and in revealing some adnexal masses, particularly if the patient's urinary bladder is empty. Transabdominal scanning provides a better overview of pelvic structures, which is helpful for less experienced users, as well as revealing structures beyond the relatively shallower field of view afforded by the transvaginal transducer. A prudent approach is to use both scan routes when the initial scanning does not definitively answer the clinical question at hand. In no case should the absence of abnormal sonographic findings cause the physician to ignore physical findings of serious disease.

Transabdominal Scanning Technique

Transabdominal ultrasound of the patient with an early pregnancy, like gynecologic ultrasound in the nonpregnant patient, requires a distended urinary bladder. The filled urinary bladder acts as a near perfect acoustic window for the transmission of ultrasound waves, displacing bowel loops from the pelvis (Fig. 2–86). An inadequately filled urinary bladder is one of the most common causes of an inadequate transabdominal pelvic ultrasound. Urine is often obtained for analysis and pregnancy testing when the patient first presents to the emergency department, and the pelvic examination is best performed with an empty bladder;

therefore, the need for bladder filling is extremely common. In cases of some urgency, direct filling is accomplished by means of a Foley catheter (300 to 500 mL of fluid can be infused) or, in more leisurely circumstances, by intravenous or oral routes. If a Foley catheter is used, the physician should avoid instilling air into the bladder, because air causes sound waves to be reflected and scattered, thus obscuring the view.

Ordinarily, the examination is begun with a 3.5-MHz transducer placed just above the pubic symphysis, which is an easily palpable, ultrasound reflective structure. Starting in the midline, both the sagittal and (after rotating the probe 90 degrees) the transverse views of the anechoic bladder should be immediately visible. Some degree of cephalad angulation of the probe enhances visualization of the uterine fundus posterior to the bladder. The transducer may be angulated and moved off the mid-line for optimal visualization of the additional structures within the pelvis. Identification of sonographic signs of pregnancy includes the presence of a gestational (chorionic) sac, fetal pole,

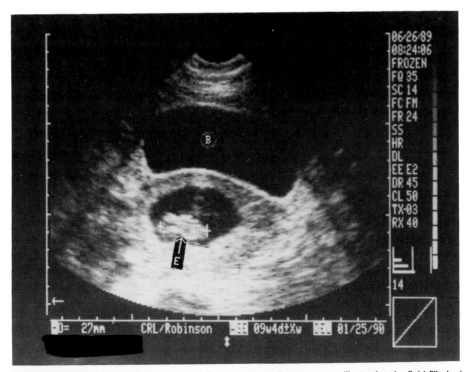

Figure 2–86. Transabdominal transverse image of a 9.5-week intrauterine pregnancy illustrating the fluid-filled urinary bladder (B) overlying the pregnant uterus and acting as an acoustic window. The embryo (E), with a crown–rump length of 27 mm, is seen between the calipers. (Courtesy of Mark Deutchman, MD.)

and fetal cardiac activity. Cardiac activity and embryonic size should be carefully identified and documented. Both normal and abnormal structures that are suspected on physical examination may often be clarified by performing a digital vaginal examination while simultaneously scanning. Demonstration of the chorionic sac and, particularly, fetal cardiac activity to the patient routinely provides excellent rapport between the examiner and the patient and often provides a gratifying therapeutic benefit as well. Hard-copy documentation of the fetal heart rate can be made by using M-mode imaging (Fig. 2–87).

Transvaginal Scanning Technique

Transvaginal scanning should be preceded by a bimanual pelvic examination. These examinations complement one another, and the sonographic examination is expedited by knowing about the relative position of the uterus, palpable masses, a stool-filled rectum, etc. The transvaginal ultrasound examination may also be preceded by a transabdominal scan in order to avoid missing structures that are at the pelvic brim, out of the range of the transvaginal transducer's depth of field. Although it is true that transvaginal scanning does not require the presence of a full urinary bladder, the presence of some urine in the bladder actually aids in the process by providing a landmark to help orient the examiner.

Performing a transvaginal scan involves the following steps:

1. Preliminary pelvic examination to find palpable masses; to determine the size, shape, and position of the uterus; and to find any areas of tenderness. Any tampon should be removed.
2. A transabdominal scan may be performed to obtain an overview of any obvious findings. If the patient is obese or her bladder is empty, findings may be limited. Examining the upper abdomen may reveal free fluid in the subhepatic area in cases of intraabdominal hemorrhage.
3. Counseling the patient about the examination and obtaining verbal consent.
4. The probe must be clean and the probe tip covered with a small amount of conductive gel; vaginal secretions must be kept from touching the shaft of the transducer. Nonlu-

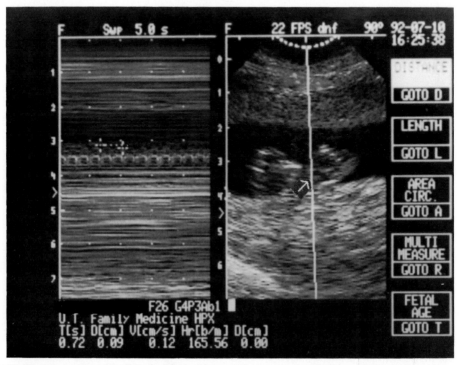

Figure 2–87. M-mode tracing on the left of a 10-week intrauterine pregnancy. The M-mode locator beam is seen passing through the area of the fetal heart on the right (*arrow*). (Courtesy of Mark Deutchman, MD.)

bricated plain end latex condoms work well for this. A latex examining glove is usually satisfactory.

5. The examiner, wearing an examination glove, applies lubricating gel to the covered tip of the probe and gently inserts it into the vagina.

6. The scan is performed using a series of sagittal (Fig. 2–88), coronal (Fig. 2–89), and oblique approaches with the transducer at varying depths of penetration. Important findings and areas of tenderness are documented with labeled, hard-copy images.

The examination should include a search for the uterus, which may be deviated to one side or the other, and viewing the uterus in sagittal, coronal, and oblique planes. Note that the transverse plane does not exist in transvaginal scanning because the probe can never be truly oriented transversely to the long axis of the patient's body. The bladder, which usually contains a small amount of urine even in patients who have just voided, can be used to help in spatial orientation. The ovaries should also be examined. In patients who have not had pelvic surgery and in whom the uterus is small, the

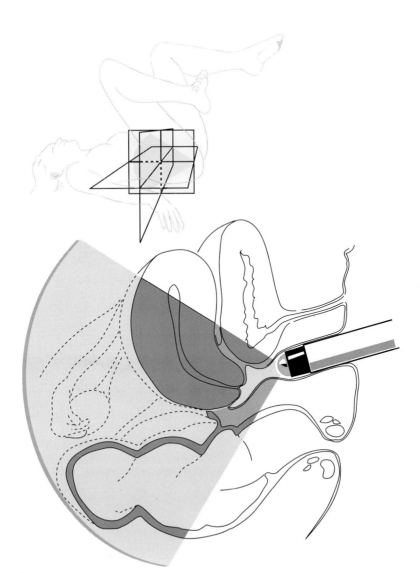

Figure 2–88. Sagittal plane. Transvaginal scanning in the sagittal or longitudinal plane is accomplished by pointing the marker dot anteriorly. The left side of the screen corresponds with the anterior abdominal wall.

ovaries are usually seen lying adjacent to the iliac vessels, which serve as good landmarks in locating the ovaries. The endometrial echo and thickness should be evaluated and the uterine contents should be thoroughly screened (Figs. 2–86, 2–90, 2–92, 2–93, 2–94, and 2–95), noting the size and shape of any fluid-filled areas, the presence and appearance of a chorionic sac, the quality of the echogenic chorionic ring, and the contents of the chorionic sac, including the yolk sac and embryo. A crown–rump measurement of the embryo is taken, and the presence or absence of cardiac activity is explicitly noted. A mean chorionic sac diameter is measured as described below. The presence of fluid or masses in the cul-de-sac should be documented, and any areas of tenderness should be correlated with the underlying structures.

Orientation of the sonographic image during transvaginal scanning can be made with the transducer–skin interface either at the top of the picture or at the bottom, depending on the examiner's preference (Fig. 2–91A and B). Regardless, the patient's left side appears on the right side of the screen in the standard coronal image. Images are labeled with the date, the patient's name, the orientation of the image, and the significant findings.

After completion of the examination, the probe is withdrawn, the cover and examining glove are discarded as contaminated waste, and the probe is cleaned according to the manufacturer's specifications.

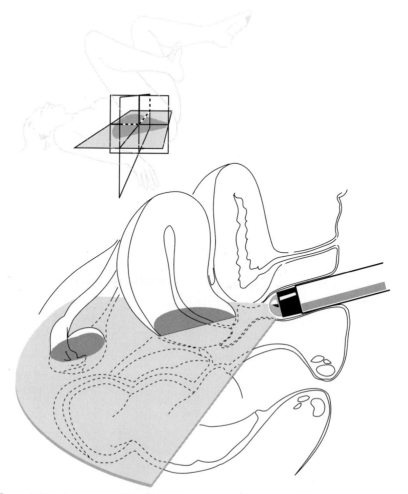

Figure 2–89. Coronal plane. Transvaginal scanning in the coronal plane is accomplished by pointing the marker dot toward the patient's right side.

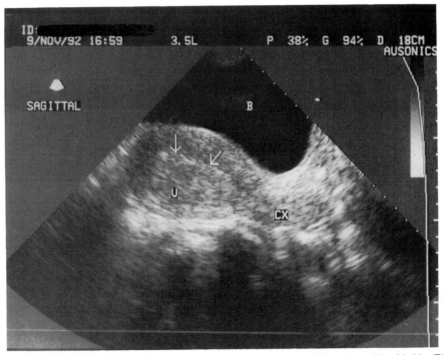

Figure 2–90. A midline sagittal transabdominal scan of the uterus (U) and cervix (CX), with overlying bladder (B) illustrating the endometrial echo (*arrows*). (Courtesy of Mark Deutchman, MD.)

NORMAL FINDINGS IN EARLY PREGNANCY

The earliest sonographic finding of a normal intrauterine pregnancy is a small, sonolucent area within the uterine cavity surrounded by a bright echogenic ring (Fig. 2–92). This is the chorionic sac, also called a gestational sac. When first visible, the chorionic sac contains no identifiable structures. By the time the mean diameter of the chorionic sac reaches 5 to 8 mm, the first distinct embryonic structure, the yolk sac, may be detectable, depending on the resolution of the ultrasound equipment being used (Fig. 2–93). By the end of the sixth menstrual week, the mean diameter of the chorionic sac grows by a millimeter a day, the yolk sac appears, and embryonic cardiac activity may be seen between the yolk sac and the wall of the chorionic sac even before an embryo is measurable (Fig. 2–94). At this point, the embryo is much smaller than the yolk sac and is surrounded by a very tiny amniotic membrane. This complex, located between the yolk sac and the chorionic wall, is termed the *fetal pole* (Figs. 2–95A and B). Most of the chorionic sac is filled by the extraembryonic

celom. The yolk sac is an extraamniotic structure. The amnion and chorion do not completely fuse until about 14 weeks, obliterating the extraembryonic celom. The embryo grows by about 1 mm per day in crown–rump length, and by the end of the seventh menstrual week measures 5 to 10 mm and exhibits cardiac motion on both transvaginal and transabdominal scanning. Transvaginal scanning is more sensitive in defining these early structures (Fig. 2–95).

Formulas for early pregnancy dating based on sonographic findings include:

1. Menstrual age in days equal 30 plus the mean sac diameter in millimeters. Mean sac diameter is calculated by measuring the chorionic sac in three planes, adding the measurements, and dividing by three (Fig. 2–96 A and B).
2. Menstrual age in weeks equals crown–rump length in centimeters plus 6.5. It is important when taking a crown–rump length measurement to avoid including the yolk sac in this measurement (Fig. 2–97). Measurement of the mean sac diameter before an embryo is visible or crown–rump length once an em-

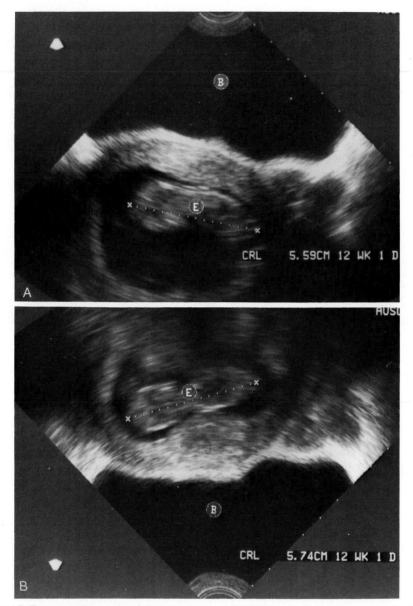

Figure 2–91. *A* and *B*, Transvaginal scan of a 12-week pregnancy with transducer–skin interface located at the top of the image in *A* and at the bottom in *B*. A small amount of urine in the maternal bladder (B) can help orient the examiner (E, embryo). (Courtesy of Mark Deutchman, MD.)

bryo appears is important. If the emergency department examination is the patient's first, it will be relied on for purposes of pregnancy dating and growth assessment, particularly if the patient is lost to follow-up for several weeks. If the emergency department examination is not the first, data are needed to compare with previous measurements in order to assess growth and the prognosis of the pregnancy.

The gold standard for the diagnosis of a living intrauterine pregnancy is the visualization of embryonic cardiac activity. This may be seen as early as 41 to 43 menstrual days (6 weeks) or when the mean sac diameter is 12 to 16 mm, depending on the resolution of the equipment and the skill of the examiner. In one study of patients who had known conception dates, transvaginal scanning revealed embryonic cardiac motion by 32 days postconception, which cor-

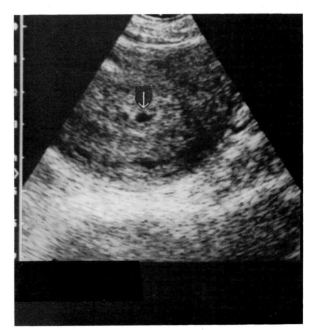

Figure 2-92. The earliest sonographic finding of a normal intrauterine pregnancy is a very small, sonolucent area (*arrow*) within the uterine cavity surrounded by a brighter, more echogenic area. This chorionic sac, or gestational sac, in this case measures only a few millimeters in diameter. No yolk sac or embryo is yet visible. (Courtesy of Mark Deutchman, MD.)

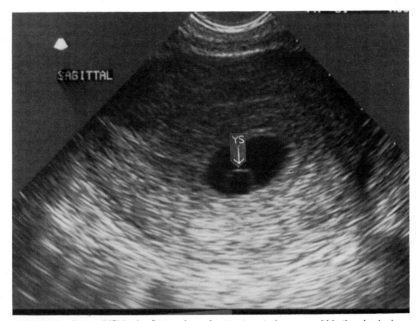

Figure 2-93. This spherical yolk sac (YS) is the first embryonic structure to be seen within the chorionic sac. (Courtesy of Mark Deutchman, MD)

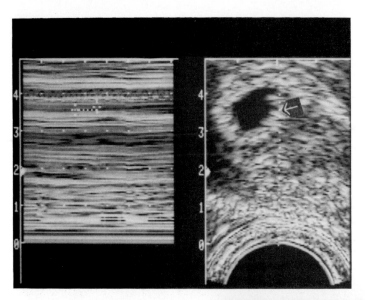

Figure 2–94. Early embryonic cardiac activity as documented by M-mode on the left. On the right, the M-mode beam is seen passing through the fetal pole (*arrow*) at the edge of the chorionic sac. (Courtesy of Mark Deutchman, MD.)

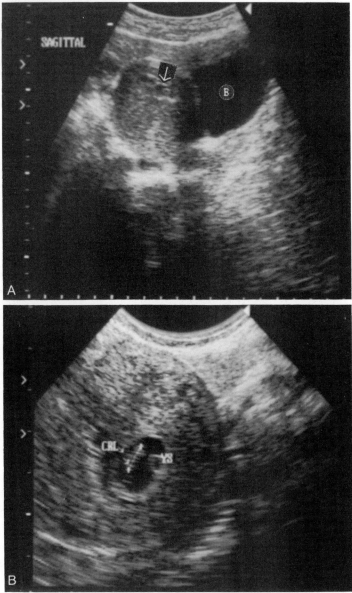

Figure 2–95. *A* and *B*, *A*, A transabdominal sagittal scan showing vague intrauterine findings (*arrow*). B, bladder. *B*, A transvaginal scan of the same patient on the same day demonstrating an embryo with crown–rump length (CRL) measured and yolk sac (YS) visible. Cardiac activity was visible in this 7-mm embryo, corresponding to 7+ weeks. This illustrates the power of transvaginal scanning. (Courtesy of Mark Deutchman, MD.)

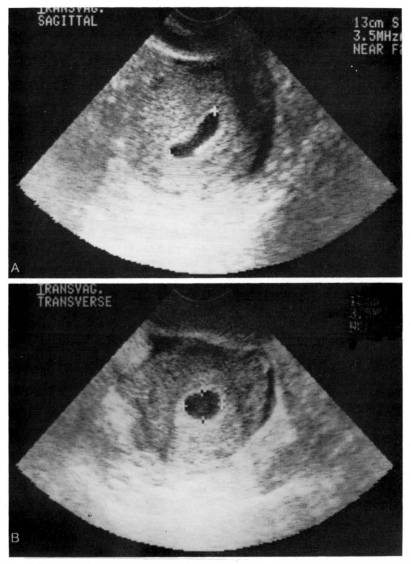

Figure 2–96. *A* and *B*, The mean diameter of the chorionic sac is calculated by measuring in three planes, adding the measurements, and dividing by three. The menstrual age in days equals 30 plus the mean sac diameter in millimeters. (Courtesy of Mark Deutchman, MD.)

responds to about 46 days from the expected date of the last normal menstrual period. Embryonic cardiac activity was never seen before 26 days postconception, corresponding to about 40 days (5.7 weeks) since the expected last normal menstrual period. During the eighth menstrual week and thereafter, the embryo is clearly identifiable by both transvaginal and transabdominal scanning (Tables 2–4 to 2–6).

ECTOPIC PREGNANCY

Ectopic pregnancy can be effectively ruled out by the emergency physician if the sonographic examination identifies the single finding of an intrauterine pregnancy. The only exception to this rule is simultaneous intrauterine and extrauterine pregnancy: heterotopic pregnancy. This rarity occurs in 1 in 30,000 low-risk pregnancies or up to 1 in 7000 pregnancies involving assisted reproductive technology. Sonography can provide a wealth of information depending on the skill of the examiner, time available, and quality of equipment used, but the diagnostic power to quickly identify a pregnancy as intrauterine makes it the primary tool in the investigation of a suspected ectopic pregnancy.

Eight possible categories of intrauterine and

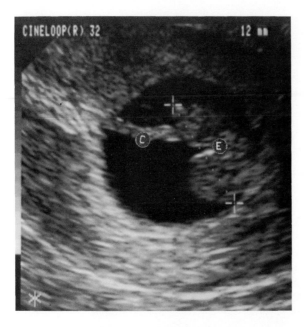

Figure 2–97. Transvaginal scan of a 7.7-week intrauterine pregnancy showing the embryo (E) and umbilical cord (C). The embryo's crown–rump length is 12 mm and is shown between the calipers. (Courtesy of Mark Deutchman, MD.)

extrauterine findings in the patient without a visible intrauterine pregnancy are described below.

1. Confirmed Ectopic Pregnancy. This implies visualization of an empty uterus and a live (fetal heart motion) embryo outside the uterus (Fig. 2–98). This finding is uncommon (less than 25% of patients with transvaginal scanning and 10% when the transabdominal approach is used). It should be clear, therefore, that mistaking the location of fetal heart motion is a grave error.

2. Highly Likely Ectopic Pregnancy. This

category is reserved for those patients in whom the uterus appears empty, but in whom ancillary findings of an ectopic pregnancy are present. The findings include an echogenic pelvic mass (Fig. 2–99) or free pelvic fluid (Fig. 2–100). The sonographic appearance of ectopic pregnancy is usually complex, containing both echogenic and sonolucent components. Blood may account for a significant portion of the volume of an ectopic pregnancy and has a highly variable sonographic appearance, depending on whether it is fresh active bleeding, clotted, or old partly liquefied blood. Examination of

Table 2–4. CONSERVATIVE DISCRIMINATORY SONOGRAPHIC AND hCG LANDMARKS

Weeks Since Last Normal Menses	Transabdominal Landmarks	Transvaginal Landmarks	Serum hCG value, mIU per mL* IRP	2nd I.S.
5 weeks	5- to 8-mm chorionic sac	5- to 8-mm chorionic sac with or without yolk sac	1,800	900
6 weeks	Yolk sac when chorionic sac is >20 mm	16-mm chorionic sac, with yolk sac and 5-mm embryo	7,200	3,800
7 weeks	5- to 10-mm embryo with heartbeat, in 25-mm chorionic sac	5- to 10-mm embryo with heartbeat, in 25-mm chorionic sac	21,000	13,200

hCG=human chorionic gonadotropin.
*The standards given are those of the World Health Organization 2nd International Standard (WHO 2nd I.S.) and the first and second International Reference Preparations (IRP).
From Deutchman ME: Advances in the diagnosis of first-trimester pregnancy problems. Am Fam Physician 1991;44(suppl):16S.

Table 2–5. TRANSABDOMINAL AND TRANSVAGINAL SCANNING

	Transabdominal	Transvaginal
Field	Wider field	Narrow field
Orientation	Orientation simple	Orientation complex
Patient Preparation	Full bladder mandatory	Empty bladder preferred
Comfort	Minimal bladder discomfort	Minimal probe discomfort
Patient acceptance	Familiar, accepted	Less familiar
Focal length	Longer focal length	Shorter focal length
Resolution	Lower resolution	Higher resolution
Frequency	3.5–5 MHz	5–7.5 MHz
Requirement	Gel required	Gel and sheath required
Probe preparation	Each use	Disinfected after each use
Scanning planes	Sagittal, transverse, and oblique	Sagittal, coronal, oblique
Labeling requirement	Important	More important

Table 2–6. ESSENTIAL INFORMATION IN A NONEMERGENT FIRST TRIMESTER ULTRASOUND REPORT

1. General size and shape of the uterus and its contents
2. Adnexal structures visible
3. Comment on presence or absence of cul-de-sac fluid
4. Specific location of the chorionic sac: intrauterine or extrauterine, and if intrauterine, where in the uterus
5. Mean chorionic sac diameter (MSD), obtained by an average of three measurements taken in perpendicular planes and correlated with menstrual gestational age by a standard technique, such as by this formula:

$$MSD \text{ (mm)} + 30 = GA \text{ (days)} \pm 4 \text{ days}$$

6. Chorionic sac number and condition of echogenic ring (chorionic villi)
7. Contents of the chorionic sac:
   a. Embryo with crown–rump measurement compared with standard tables to calculate gestational age. An approximation of gestational age from crown–rump length (CRL) can be obtained using this formula:

$$CRL \text{ (cm)} + 6.5 = \text{menstrual age (weeks)}$$

   b. Presence or absence of embryonic cardiac motion (can be documented with M-mode)
   c. Yolk sac size, shape, and appearance
8. Findings should be compared with those of any previous scans, and the growth of the chorionic sac and the embryo should be noted as normal or not. Chorionic sac mean diameters increase at the rate of 1.1 mm per day. Embryos grow about 1 mm per day.

From Deutchman ME: Advances in the diagnosis of first-trimester pregnancy problems. Am Fam Physician 1991; 44(suppl):26S.

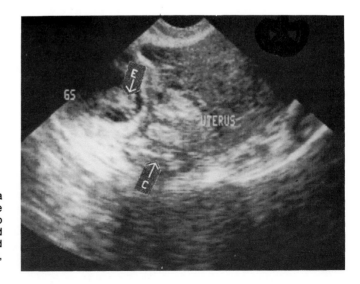

Figure 2–98. Coronal transvaginal scan of a confirmed ectopic pregnancy. The figure shows the ectopic pregnancy, labeled GS, to the right of the uterus, behind which are blood clots (C). The extrauterine embryo (E) showed cardiac motion. (Courtesy of Mark Deutchman, MD.)

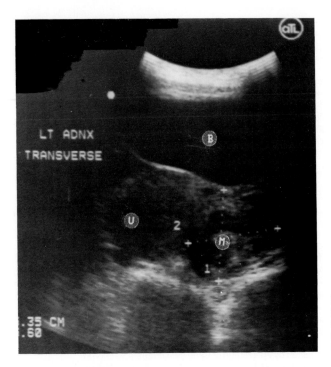

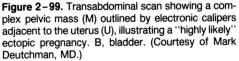

Figure 2–99. Transabdominal scan showing a complex pelvic mass (M) outlined by electronic calipers adjacent to the uterus (U), illustrating a "highly likely" ectopic pregnancy. B, bladder. (Courtesy of Mark Deutchman, MD.)

the patient's right upper quadrant is also important because blood may pool in the subhepatic area rather than in the pelvis, depending on the patient's position and the location of the ectopic pregnancy (Fig. 2–101). The risk of ectopic pregnancy depends on the particular combination of ancillary findings and is listed in Table 2–7.

3. Very Early Normal Pregnancy. This implies that the patient in fact has an intrauterine pregnancy but is prior to the time that it is expected to be visualized on ultrasound (see Fig. 2–92). Although improved equipment has increased the sensitivity in detecting pregnancy, the gestational (chorionic) sac is not visible by transabdominal ultrasound before the fifth

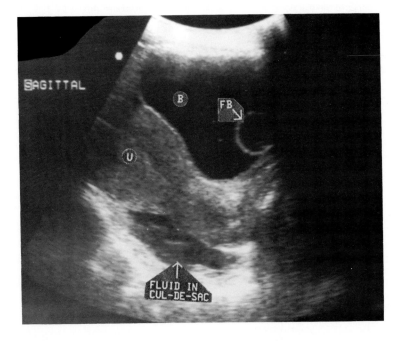

Figure 2–100. A sagittal transabdominal scan showing a large amount of free fluid behind the uterus in a case of ruptured ectopic pregnancy. The urinary bladder (B) and the Foley catheter balloon (FB) are seen above the uterus (U). (Courtesy of Mark Deutchman, MD.)

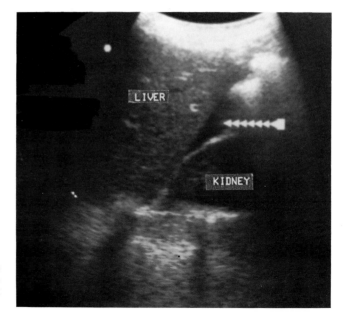

Figure 2–101. Fluid in the subhepatic area of the right upper quadrant (*arrows*) in a case of ruptured ectopic pregnancy. (Courtesy of Mark Deutchman, MD.)

menstrual week and cardiac activity may not be discernible until the seventh menstrual week. Although the transvaginal technique improves these sensitivities by up to 1 week (see Fig. 2–95), it is clear that many very early pregnancies will still not be sonographically apparent. Clearly, such patients would not be expected to be able to exhibit any of the ancillary findings of ectopic pregnancy, and it may be impossible to establish — by any technique — that the pregnancy is intrauterine as opposed to ectopic. With the almost-routine use of sensitive pregnancy tests on women of childbearing age, incidentally pregnant patients are being identified with increasing frequency in the emergency department. All such cases would require follow-up with clinical examination and possibly serial ultrasound or serum hormone testing to ascertain that the pregnancy is in fact intrauterine.

4. Occult Unruptured Ectopic Pregnancy. This implies that an early ectopic pregnancy does in fact exist, but that there are no ancillary signs present. A subset of this group in fact demonstrates the pseudo sac in the uterus, which is illustrated in Figure 2–102. Pseudo sac refers to a sonolucent fluid collection within the uterus that occurs with some ectopic pregnancies. Pseudo sacs characteristically lack the bright echogenic ring found in a true gestational (chorionic) sac and do not contain a yolk sac or fetal pole. Nonetheless, the possibility of misidentifying this structure as a true gestational sac underscores the importance of recognizing a typical fetal pole and preferably fetal heart motion as the gold standard for the diagnosis of intrauterine pregnancy. The management when a gestational sac cannot be confirmed is individualized and may include either inpatient or out-

Table 2–7. RISK OF ECTOPIC PREGNANCY IN PATIENTS WITH POSITIVE hCG AND EMPTY UTERUS ON TRANSABDOMINAL ULTRASOUND

Ancillary Findings	Risk of Ectopic Pregnancy (%)
Any free fluid	20
Echogenic mass	71
Moderate/large fluid	95
Echogenic mass with fluid	100
No ancillary findings	20

From Mahony BS, Filly RA, Nyberg DA, Callen PW: Sonographic evaluation of ectopic pregnancy. J Ultrasound Med 1985;4:221–228.

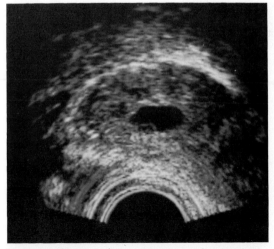

Figure 2–102. Coronal transvaginal scan of a uterus containing a "pseudo sac" in a patient who had an ectopic pregnancy. The pseudo sac is not surrounded by an echogenic chorionic ring. (Courtesy of Mark Deutchman, MD.)

patient follow-up with serial ultrasound, serum hormone testing (as described below), or laparoscopy.

5. Complete or Incomplete Spontaneous Abortion (Miscarriage). In such cases, ultrasound examination reveals an empty uterus or one containing atypical echogenic or sonolucent findings. If the thickness of the uterine contents exceeds 5 mm, retained tissue is highly likely (Fig. 2–103). The uterus may be tender due to the miscarriage, and these patients require follow-up and perhaps diagnostic and therapeutic curettage to eventually establish the diagnosis.

From an emergency physician's standpoint, the use of diagnostic ultrasound yields a definitive diagnosis in the emergency department in the large majority of patients who have a living intrauterine pregnancy and yields a presumptive diagnosis in those at high risk for ectopic pregnancy. The remainder of patients who are at low risk with an absence of ancillary findings and who are clinically stable receive individualized attention and follow-up with appropriate consultation. Figure 2–104 summarizes the sonographic approach to patients clinically suspected of having an ectopic pregnancy.

OTHER EMERGENCY DEPARTMENT PROBLEMS IN EARLY PREGNANCY

Three additional conditions may become apparent when a first trimester patient with pelvic pain or bleeding is scanned. Although these conditions do not represent true, immediate emergencies, they all require early follow-up.

6. Dead Embryo. The embryonic heart rate is about 100 beats per minute (bpm) when first visible, rises sharply to about 170 bpm at 9 weeks, and then declines gradually to the familiar 120 to 160 bpm range. Although embryonic cardiac motion can sometimes be seen between the yolk sac and the wall of the chorionic sac during the sixth menstrual week (Figs. 2–87 and 2–94), the absence of cardiac motion at this point is not a definitive sign of embryonic demise. The diagnosis of embryonic demise is ap-

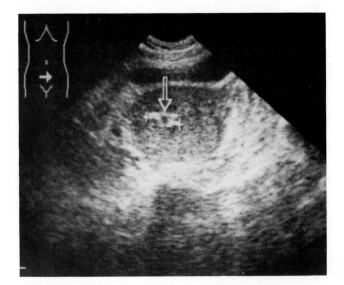

Figure 2–103. Transabdominal transverse scan of a uterus containing a 23-mm echogenic area (*arrow*), indicating retained tissue. (Courtesy of Mark Deutchman, MD.)

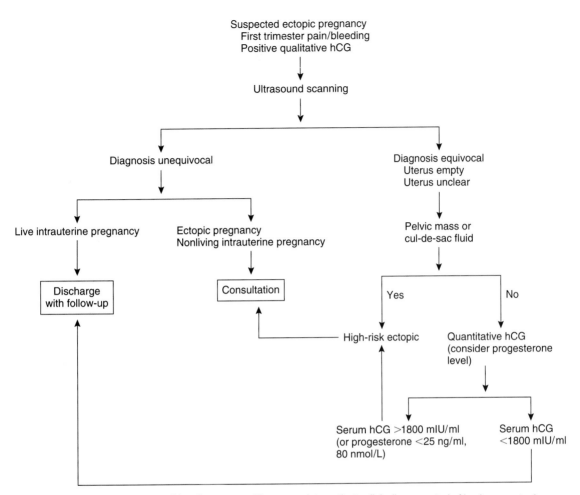

Figure 2–104. Flowchart summarizing the sonographic approach to patients clinically suspected of having an ectopic pregnancy.

propriate if an embryo with a crown–rump length of at least 5 mm exhibits no cardiac motion during a period of continuous observation (Fig. 2–105). In the absence of heavy vaginal bleeding, the diagnosis and treatment of embryonic demise does not constitute an emergency by itself. Therefore, it is quite appropriate to offer such patients follow-up and reevaluation within a few days in order to confirm this diagnosis.

7. Embryonic Resorption/Blighted Ovum. The diagnosis of embryonic resorption or blighted ovum is made sonographically when a chorionic sac is present of sufficient size that an embryo should be visible, but none is found (Fig. 2–106). The mean diameter of a chorionic sac, which must contain an embryo, is about 16 mm when viewed transvaginally. In addition to the absence of a normal embryo, other ancillary

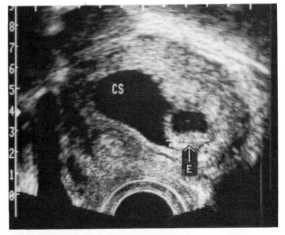

Figure 2–105. Coronal transvaginal scan of a uterus containing a dead embryo (E) located between the electronic calipers. No cardiac motion was seen, despite the crown–rump length of 1.6 cm, corresponding to 8+ weeks. CS, chorionic sac. (Courtesy of Mark Deutchman, MD.)

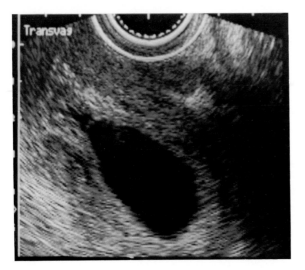

Figure 2–106. Transvaginal scan of an "empty" chorionic sac in a case of embryonic resorption, also known as blighted ovum. (Courtesy of Mark Deutchman, MD.)

findings often help make this diagnosis sonographically. These include a chorionic sac that has lost its bright echogenic ring, one that appears misshapen, location low in the uterus rather than in the fundus, and the presence of debris that represents a degenerated or partly reabsorbed embryo. In the past, such cases were thought to represent pregnancies in which an embryo never developed. However, current thinking based on high-resolution scanning indicates that the embryo dies at an early point in such pregnancies and degenerates or is absorbed. As with embryonic demise, such cases

do not demand emergency treatment except when bleeding is severe. Therefore, in doubtful cases, a follow-up examination is entirely appropriate.

8. Hydatidiform Mole/Trophoblastic Disease. The sonographic hallmarks of first trimester hydatidiform molar pregnancy are a snowstorm appearance of the uterine contents (Fig. 2–107), often with some scattered, larger sonolucent areas, and the associated theca lutein ovarian cysts, which may reach a very large size. Such patients may present with bleeding, but passing the grape-like vesicles (as they are often

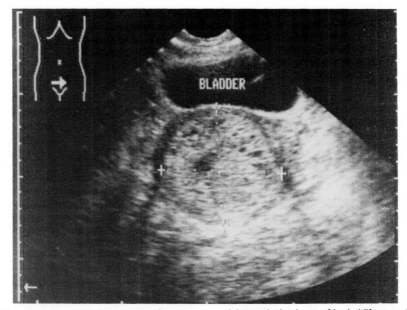

Figure 2–107. Transabdominal transverse scan of a uterus containing typical echoes of hydatidiform mole. (Courtesy of Mark Deutchman, MD.)

described in obstetrics textbooks) is not common during the first trimester. Although stable patients with this diagnosis do not require emergency hospital admission, prompt arrangement of follow-up for the performance of a suction dilatation and curettage (D & C) within the next few days is mandatory because of the possibility of malignant degeneration into choriocarcinoma. The theca lutein cysts can be expected to resolve spontaneously.

Sonographic Guidance of Clinical Procedures

There are two emergent gynecologic procedures in which diagnostic ultrasound can be of significant benefit: culdocentesis and suction curettage.

Culdocentesis

Although the increasing availability of diagnostic ultrasound and sensitive urine and serum hormone testing has almost obviated the need for culdocentesis in many institutions, there remain certain clinical situations where the procedure is useful. For example, the ultrasound finding of significant pelvic fluid in a patient with abdominal pain may raise the issue of ruptured ovarian cyst versus ruptured ectopic pregnancy. In some cases, the differentiation between the two may depend on the quality of the fluid that is aspirated from the culdocentesis. The hemoperitoneum seen from ruptured ectopic pregnancy is ordinarily distinguished from the thinner, more serous fluid of a ruptured ovarian cyst. Although it is traditionally done in a blind fashion, culdocentesis can be facilitated by visualizing the fluid pocket transabdominally while the aspirating needle is advanced into the cul-de-sac. A 20- or 21-gauge spinal needle usually can be clearly seen sonographically as it enters the fluid-filled pouch.

Suction Curettage

Although suction curettage of incomplete spontaneous abortions is now commonly performed as an outpatient procedure, it is not usually performed by emergency physicians except in truly emergent settings or when a specialty consultation is not available. Transabdominal ultrasound scanning performed simultaneously with suction curettage has the advantage of identifying the fundus of the uterus and the character and volume of the remaining uterine content. Because the curettage instruments — both the ring forceps and the suction curette — have a bright echogenic appearance, they can be visualized within the uterine fundus, decreasing the risk of inadvertent perforation.

Clinical Considerations

Although ultrasonography is a very powerful tool in the diagnosis of first trimester pregnancy problems, the hand-held Doppler probe is a simpler, less expensive device that can be employed first. When a fetal heartbeat is heard with the Doppler probe, pregnancy loss has been ruled out, and ectopic pregnancy is much less likely because Doppler fetal heart tones are not heard until 9 or 10 weeks, and most ectopic pregnancies become symptomatic before that time. The possibility of hearing fetal heart tones with a hand-held Doppler probe is dramatically increased when the Doppler transducer is aimed directly at the uterine fundus during a bimanual pelvic examination; the fundus is identified and lifted up with the examiner's vaginal hand, while the Doppler transducer is aimed with the examiner's abdominal hand.

Serum hormone testing can be very helpful in equivocal cases or may constitute a first-line diagnostic test in emergency departments where ultrasound is not available. The correlation between menstrual date, the ultrasound landmarks, and expected hCG values is given in Table 2–4. A serum progesterone less than 25 ng/mL or a quantitative serum hCG over 1800 MIU/mL with an empty or equivocal uterus on ultrasound places the patient in a high-risk group for ectopic pregnancy and constitutes a reason for prompt consultation and referral. The cost of quantitative hCG and progesterone testing often exceeds that of an ultrasound scan, and the results are seldom immediately available. Such testing can be very helpful in equivocal cases or as a screen for determining which patients need to be recalled for sonographic evaluation when ultrasonography was not performed at the time of initial presentation.

Both physicians and patients suspect that pain (or bleeding) during the first trimester of pregnancy is most likely a complication of the pregnancy. When the diagnostic ultrasound evaluation determines that the pregnancy is intrauterine, the search for other causes of the patient's symptoms can sometimes be facilitated by the ultrasound examination. Pelvic inflammatory disease, ruptured ovarian cyst, appendicitis, adnexal torsion, and urolithiasis are among the other considerations that may be occasionally suggested by ultrasound findings.

The use of sonography in early pregnancy often provides the patient with an immediate, definitive diagnosis. This can aid greatly in counseling her about the type and urgency of follow-up needed and can offer a prognosis for the continuation of the pregnancy. It is also important to counsel patients in whom an intrauterine heartbeat has been seen that miscarriage is still possible. In fact, the risk of miscarriage is up to 16% when the pregnancy is 8 menstrual weeks or less. This risk drops to 2 to 4% after 12 weeks.

Subchorionic hemorrhage may be seen as a crescent-shaped, sonolucent area adjacent to the chorionic sac. The location is more important than the size (Fig. 2–108). Hemorrhages that undermine the placental implantation site are most likely to cause miscarriage. A subchorionic hemorrhage should not be mistaken for a twin sac. The diagnosis of twins should be reserved for cases in which two chorionic sacs, two yolk sacs, and two embryos are seen. Seventy percent of twins diagnosed in the first trimester are singletons at term.

Corpus luteum cysts are common incidental findings that should not be mistaken for an ectopic or heterotopic pregnancy. These cysts can occasionally cause significant adnexal pain (Fig. 2–109). Cystic and other pelvic masses are considered more fully in Chapter 3, "Gynecologic Applications."

Conclusion and Summary

Diagnostic ultrasound is an indispensable tool in the emergency department management of suspected ectopic pregnancy. When used as the first diagnostic test in problem first trimester patients, it offers the opportunity to make an immediate definitive diagnosis in a large percentage of cases and offers prognostic information and therapeutic guidance in most of the remainder of cases. The addition of transvaginal sonography has further enhanced the sensitivity of the technique, but there remains a subset of patients with early pregnancy (4 to 6 weeks) in whom the emergency department diagnosis is not possible and for whom referral for clinical, sonographic, or hormonal follow-up is needed.

COMMON ERRORS IN EMERGENCY PELVIC SCANNING

1. Failure to ensure a very full bladder when performing transabdominal scanning
2. Overinterpreting a small amount of fluid in the cul-de-sac as evidence of leakage from

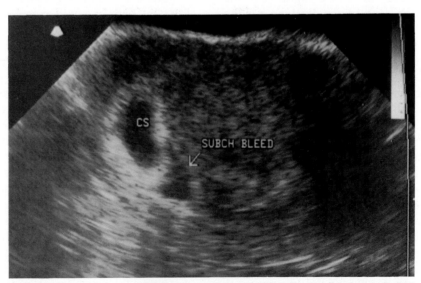

Figure 2–108. Transvaginal scan of uterus containing a chorionic sac (CS) with an adjacent subchorionic hemorrhage (SUBCH BLEED). (Courtesy of Mark Deutchman, MD.)

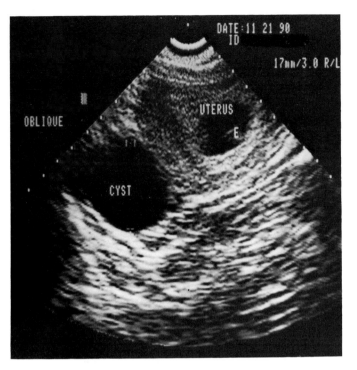

Figure 2-109. Oblique transabdominal scan shows a uterus that contains a chorionic sac and embryo (E) and adjacent 4.2-cm cyst. This is a typical appearance of a corpus luteum cyst accompanying a normal intrauterine pregnancy.

an ectopic pregnancy or from an ovarian cyst

3. Identifying a large ovarian cyst as urinary bladder

4. Assuming that a normal-appearing gestational sac with a viable embryo is necessarily intrauterine

5. Misdiagnosing an empty gestational sac of more than 2.5 cm as a normal early pregnancy

6. Mistaking a pseudo gestational sac for an intrauterine pregnancy

7. Misinterpreting the hyperechoic decidual reaction within the uterus as evidence of intrauterine pregnancy

8. Neglecting to obtain a quantitative hCG when the sonographic findings are not consistent with the dates

9. Neglecting to transabdominal scan when transvaginal scan does not explain symptoms

10. Failure to consider all eight distinct possibilities in a patient with a positive hCG but no intrauterine pregnancy on ultrasound

SELECTED READINGS

Abbott J, Emmans LS, Lowenstein SR: Ectopic pregnancy: Ten common pitfalls in diagnosis. Am J Emerg Med 1990;8:515–522.

Deutchman M: Advances in the diagnosis of first-trimester pregnancy problems. Am Fam Physician 1991;44 (suppl):15S–30S.

Graham M, Cooperberg PL: Ultrasound of interstitial pregnancy: Findings and pitfalls. J Clin Ultrasound 1979; 7:433–437.

Kurtz AB, Shlansky-Goldberg RD, Choi HY, et al: Detection of retained products of conception following spontaneous abortion in the first trimester. J Ultrasound Med 1991;10:387–395.

Maliha WE, Gonella P, Degnan EJ: Ruptured interstitial pregnancy presenting as an intrauterine pregnancy by ultrasound. Ann Emerg Med 1991;20:910–912.

Matthews CP, Coulson RB, Wild RA: Serum progesterone levels as an aid in the diagnosis of ectopic pregnancy. Obstet Gynecol 1986;68:390.

Rosenberg RD, Williamson MR: Cervical ectopic pregnancy: Avoiding pitfalls in the ultrasonographic diagnosis. J Ultrasound Med 1992;11:365–367.

Sherer DM, Abramowicz JS, Thompson HO, et al: Comparison of transabdominal and endovaginal sonographic approaches in the diagnosis of a case of cervical pregnancy successfully treated with methotrexate. J Ultrasound Med 1991;10:409–411.

Smith CB, Sakornbut EL, Dickinson LC, Bullock GL: Quantification of training in obstetrical ultrasound: A study of family practice residents. J Clin Ultrasound 1991;19:479–483.

Trolanos CA, Jobes DR, Eillison N: Ultrasound-guided cannulation of the internal jugular vein: A prospective, randomized study. Anesth Analg 1991;72:823–826.

Texts

Both general ultrasonography texts and OB/GYN ultrasonography texts have sections relevant for the emergency physician, with the OB/GYN texts more clinically oriented. The endovaginal texts are concise and worthwhile.

Callen PW: Ultrasonography in OB/GYN, 2nd ed. Philadelphia: W. B. Saunders, 1988. *A complete standard work.*

Fleischer AC, James AE: Diagnostic Sonography: Principles and Clinical Applications. Philadelphia: W. B. Saunders, 1989. *This general ultrasound text devotes approximately 50 pages to the abnormal first trimester pregnancy. There are many images with graphics (most transabdominal), all the necessary tables and graphs, and excellent, if slightly dated, references.*

Hagen-Ansert SL: Textbook of Diagnostic Ultrasonography, 3rd ed. St. Louis: C. V. Mosby, 1986. *A complete, technique-oriented review in this sonographer-edited general book.*

Tessler RN, Perella RR, Grant EG, Doherty FS: Handbook of Endovaginal Sonography. New York: Thieme, 1992. *This small, soft-cover handbook, written by radiologists, emphasizes ultrasound appearance rather than clinical correlations. Complete presentation of normal transvaginal examination; less than 10 pages on ectopic pregnancy.*

Timor-Tritsch IE, Rotten S: Transvaginal Sonography, 2nd ed. New York: Elsevier Science Publishing, 1991. *The fathers of transvaginal ultrasound cover all aspects. Very clinically oriented.*

Cardiac Applications

David Plummer, MD, and Michael Heller, MD

Two-dimensional (2-D) echocardiography is the application of ultrasound technologies to the study of the heart and great vessels. As with the stethoscope and electrocardiogram (ECG) that preceded it, but unlike the host of angiographic, hemodynamic, and radionucleotide studies that have recently become available, 2-D echocardiography is well suited to bedside emergency department use in that it is rapid, accurate, noninvasive, and allows for serial examinations. Echocardiography provides a great deal of anatomic and functional information that the physician must then interpret, based on the patient's clinical condition. In both types of examinations, the interpretation may be obvious even to the novice, such as with a large pericardial effusion, or it may be highly complex. As compared with electrocardiography, performing the 2-D echocardiographic examination is more operator-dependent, but understanding the echocardiographic anatomy is far more intuitive than interpreting the ECG's electrical vectors.

Two-dimensional echocardiography may contribute to the evaluation for many different patient presentations; these can be summarized as:

1. Hypotension (or pulselessness) of unknown cause
2. Suspicion of cardiac trauma, either blunt or penetrating
3. Ischemic heart disease
4. Disease of the great vessels
5. Suspicion of iatrogenic (procedural) complications.

Two distinct applications—the diagnosis of pericardial tamponade and the confirmation (or refutation) of electromechanical dissociation—are considered primary indications for emergency department echocardiography. Both are time-critical diagnoses and require rapid, specific intervention. Physicians recognize both conditions after a short training session. All other cardiac conditions are dealt with in Chapter 3.

CARDIAC TAMPONADE

Sonographic Considerations

It is fortunate that the sonographic detection of pericardial effusion is so straightforward, because the presence of pericardial fluid is necessary in order to establish tamponade physiology. There is often no other practical means to establish or refute the uncommon but lethal diagnosis of cardiac tamponade in the emergency department setting. Beck's triad, pulsus paradoxus, and electrical alternans are all nonspecific and late findings. Detection of pericardial fluid does not require specialized knowledge of echocardiographic cardiac anatomy, standardized cardiac windows, or much experience. Use of ultrasound to detect pericardial effusion, however, requires almost none of that; findings are usually immediate and unequivocal.

The pericardium is a dense, fibrous sac that completely encircles the heart and a few centimeters of the aorta and pulmonary artery. The dense pericardial tissue is highly echogenic and is recognized both anteriorly and posteriorly as the sonographic border of the cardiac image (Fig. 2–110). Under normal conditions, there is a small amount of fluid that serves to lubricate the space between the visceral and parietal layers of the pericardium. This fluid is usually less than 30 to 50 mL in volume and is usually not visible over the nondependent aspect of the heart. The exquisite sensitivity of ultrasound for the detection of pericardial fluid arises from the fact that the effusion appears as an anechoic space that separates the echogenic pericardium from the heart. Figure 2–111 illustrates just how obvious this appearance may be. Large pericardial effusions surround the entire heart and are visualized in virtually every view. Small effusions collect first around the more dependent and mobile ventricles. In cases with severe pericardial disease, loculated effusions may develop (Fig. 2–112) in regions that are unpredictable, but these effusions are unlikely to cause critical tamponade. Using the 3.5-MHz transducer, the physician may easily visualize all of the heart and surrounding pericardium after finding an appropriate window (one that avoids intervening lung tissue).

Echocardiographers have specifically devised several standard views for use in the echocardiographic examination. The most useful of these are presented in Chapter 3, but such de-

tailed knowledge is unnecessary for the diagnosis of pericardial effusion. Simply placing the transducer in the subcostal position just to the left of the xiphoid and aiming toward the left shoulder (marker dot pointing to the patient's right side) provides an extremely useful view. This is called the subcostal view, and it has the effect of viewing the heart from the abdomen with hepatic parenchyma often acting as an acoustic window. Chamber identification may be more difficult with this view (the right ventricle is encountered just deep to the liver and pericardium), but identifying a pericardial effusion is straightforward. Figures 2–113 and 2–114 show these characteristics and indicate the close relationship between aspects of the heart and the liver. A second easily understood view is obtained by placing the transducer parallel to the long axis of the heart. This view is obtained by placing the transducer in the left parasternal area between the second and the fourth intercostal spaces. Rotate the transducer so the marker dot is parallel to the long axis of the heart and is pointed cephalad. This view is excellent at detecting even small effusions. This long-axis view readily displays the dependent aspects of the pericardium (Figs. 2–115 and 2–116). When organized blood or fibrin is present, the effusion shows some degree of echogenicity, rather than being perfectly an-

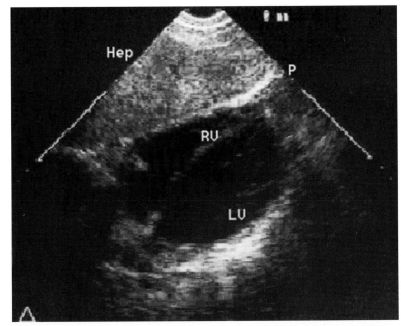

Figure 2–110. Subcostal echocardiogram. Hep, hepatic parenchyma; LV, left ventricle; RV, right ventricle.

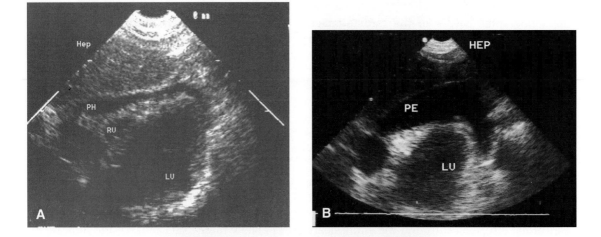

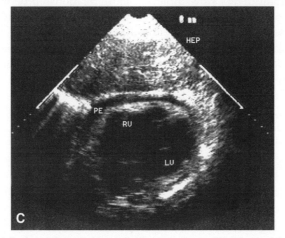

Figure 2–111. *A–C*, Subcostal echocardiogram. Hep, hepatic parenchyma; LV, left ventricle; PE, pericardial effusion; PH, pericardial hematoma (pericardial effusion); RV, right ventricle.

echoic. This may provide a clue as to the underlying cause, as in the investigation of a malignancy. Figure 2–117 shows the echogenic characteristics of organized pericardial blood. With large effusions, the heart can develop a remarkable motion as it floats within the distended pericardial sac. This is obvious when viewed in real-time sonography, but does not correlate with the presence of tamponade physiology. Several direct sonographic signs of tamponade physiology on the heart have been described, but appreciation of these may be subtle. The most important finding is a circumferential pericardial effusion with hyperdynamic heart that demonstrates diastolic collapse of the right ventricle or right atrium (Fig. 2–118). Occasionally, either intraabdominal fluid or pleural effusions may be confused with pericardial ef-

fusions. It is necessary to visualize the hyperechoic image of the pericardium to ensure that the anechoic fluid surrounding the heart is intrapericardial. The subcostal view is often most helpful, because there is no pleural reflection between the liver and the heart. A large, anechoic space visualized from the subcostal view is fluid in either free abdominal or intrapericardial space (Fig. 2–119). Intrapericardial fluid conforms to the contour of the heart, whereas free intraabdominal fluid does not.

Clinical Considerations

Before the development of bedside ultrasound, the diagnosis of acute pericardial tamponade was often difficult to establish or refute with certainty. Elevated neck veins are particularly unreliable in patients wearing an inflated

Text continued on page 133

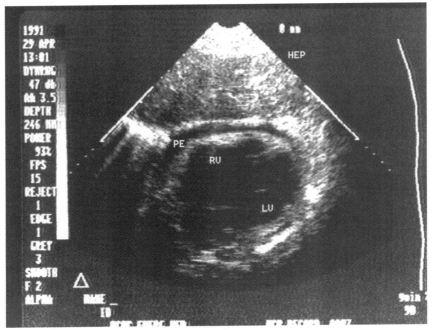

Figure 2–112. Subcostal echocardiogram in purulent pericarditis. Fib, fibrinous pericardial adhesions; LV, left ventricle; PE, pericardial effusion; RV, right ventricle. Note pericardial fluid confined to nondependent portions of pericardium.

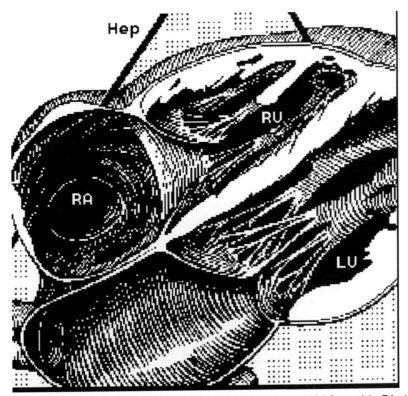

Figure 2–113. Schematic of subcostal echocardiogram. Hep, hepatic parenchyma; LV, left ventricle; RA, right atrium; RV, right ventricle.

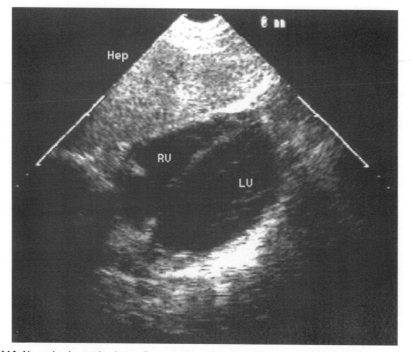

Figure 2–114. Normal subcostal echocardiogram. Hep, hepatic parenchyma; LV, left ventricle; RV, right ventricle.

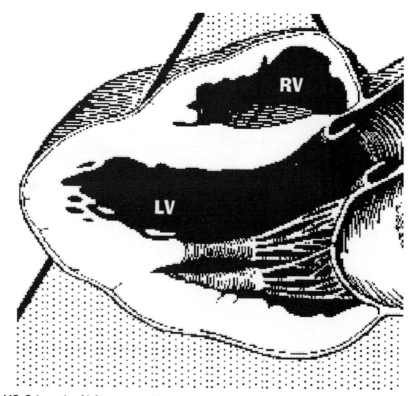

Figure 2–115. Schematic of left parasternal long-axis view echocardiogram. LV, left ventricle; RV, right ventricle.

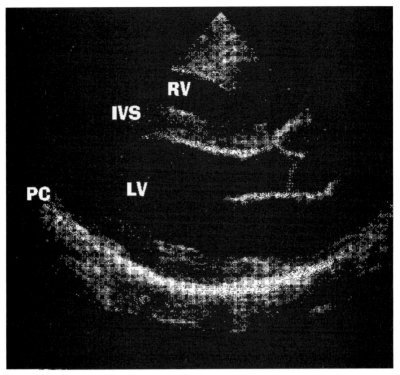

Figure 2-116. Normal left parasternal long-axis view. IVS, intraventricular septum; LV, left ventricle; PC, pericardium; RV, right ventricle.

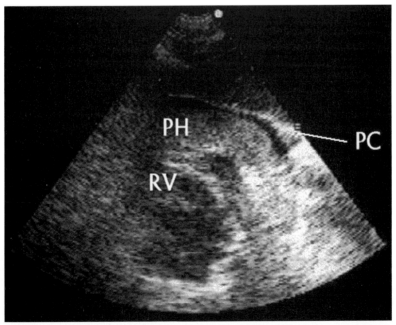

Figure 2-117. Subcostal echocardiogram of organized pericardial hematoma. Note the echogenic characteristics of organized pericardial blood. PC, pericardium; PH, pericardial hematoma; RV, right ventricle.

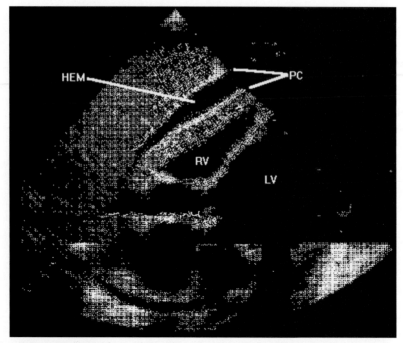

Figure 2–118. Subcostal echocardiogram in a patient with cardiac tamponade. HEM, pericardial hematoma; LV, left ventricle; PC, pericardium; RV, right ventricle.

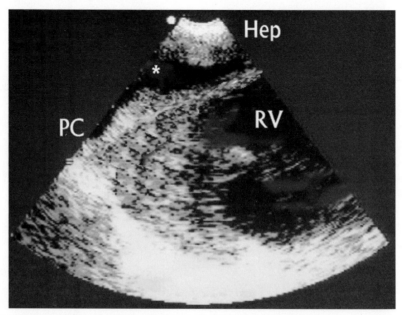

Figure 2–119. Subcostal echocardiogram showing free abdominal fluid (*asterisk*). HEP, hepatic parenchyma; PC, pericardium; RV, right ventricle. Note anechoic fluid does not follow the contour of the heart.

MAST suit, in Trendelenburg position (false positive), or hypovolemic patients without sufficient vascular volume to elevate right-sided filling pressures (false negative). Paradoxical pulse is extremely difficult to measure in a critically ill patient; it is also nonspecific. Electrical alternans, although reasonably specific for large pericardial effusions, is not sensitive for acute effusions from acute pericardial disease and is most often seen in chronic effusions without tamponade. Traditional anteroposterior chest x-ray studies usually reveal a normal cardiac silhouette with the rapid accumulation of pericardial fluid, and an enlarged cardiac silhouette is most commonly from cardiomegaly rather than from pericardial effusion. Although the absence of pericardial fluid rules out the diagnosis of pericardial tamponade, the mere presence of pericardial effusion does not determine the existence of tamponade physiology. The clinical presentation of the patient may help in this determination. A pericardial effusion found in a hemodynamically unstable young patient who sustained penetrating thoraco-abdominal injury must be considered tamponade until proven otherwise. Conversely, an effusion found in an unstable patient with known, long-standing malignancy should not be considered tamponade immediately. In borderline cases where a pericardial effusion is documented, heart catheterization or diagnostic pericardiocentesis may be required to diagnose tamponade physiology. Some special sonographic considerations relating to acute left ventricular dysfunction and possible pericardial tamponade in the setting of penetrating heart trauma are dealt with separately in Chapter 3.

ELECTROMECHANICAL DISSOCIATION

It is difficult to imagine a more straightforward use of bedside ultrasound than the documentation of electromechanical dissociation (EMD) during cardiac arrest. It is remarkable that, in the 1990s, the diagnosis of EMD is most often made by the failure to palpate a pulse while an electrical rhythm is still noted on a monitor. All physicians have encountered patients who were clearly alive and often still awake but in whom pulses could not be palpated. There are also patients who are apneic and nonresponsive

in whom a pulse cannot be palpated, yet they are still viable. There are multiple possible reasons for the failure to palpate a pulse (i.e., severe vascular disease, inadequate perfusion pressure), and if all these patients are prematurely labeled as having EMD, some potentially salvageable cases will be overlooked. Bedside emergency ultrasound can eliminate this problem in a matter of seconds.

Sonographic Considerations

The goal of the examination is simply to establish the presence of organized heart motion. Secondarily, some assessment of vigor of the cardiac contraction can be made. As with cardiac tamponade, almost any view would probably suffice, but the parasternal long-axis view with the transducer directed slightly toward the right shoulder of the patient is as favorable as any. This reveals both ventricles and particularly the left ventricle. Cardiopulmonary resuscitation (CPR) must be stopped momentarily while an assessment is made of the presence or absence of wall and valve motion. The apical view may be a very good alternative and is obtained by placing the transducer at the cardiac apex and directing it toward the right shoulder with the marker dot pointed to the patient's side. Critically ill patients often have multiple concurrent chest procedures under way at the time of the echocardiographic examination; this may leave only the subcostal approach available for cardiac imaging.

If the diagnosis of true EMD is confirmed, standard cardiac arrest protocols are followed and death is pronounced. Sonographic findings that refute this diagnosis are synchronized wall motion (especially if hyperdynamic, implying occult hypovolemia) or areas of segmental wall motion. The identification of cardiac tamponade provides a treatable alternative diagnosis. The diagnosis of tension pneumothorax can be suggested by the failure to visualize the heart due to intrapleural air. Each of these findings suggests reversible conditions.

Considerations

Studies in the past several years suggest that approximately one third of all patients thought on clinical grounds to have EMD are actually exhibiting another condition. The fact that several of these—notably, tension pneumothorax, pericardial tamponade, hypovolemia, hypoxia, hyperkalemia, pulmonary embolism, acidosis, or severe hypokinesis—are potentially reversible makes it clear that a more reliable method of confirming the diagnosis is required. Bedside ultrasonography has the advantage (as compared to hand-held Doppler study) of not only confirming or refuting the diagnosis, but suggesting what the true diagnosis is. Because true EMD appears to have a uniformly fatal prognosis, ending resuscitation efforts is usually justified. This is particularly true when means for monitoring end-tidal CO_2 production are available to confirm nonviability. The ultrasound finding of near-normal or hyperdynamic wall motion immediately suggests the presence of hypovolemia. Massive fluid resuscitation and investigation as to the site of intravascular blood loss are then undertaken. The presence of pericardial tamponade merits immediate drainage either percutaneously or perhaps more definitively through emergency thoracotomy and pericardiectomy. In cases in which wall motion and valvular motion are still noted, although inadequate to produce a pulse pressure, prompt massive inotropic therapy and perhaps balloon-pump assistance are indicated. These alternative conditions are discussed in Chapter 3. There are no data yet to suggest what subgroup of these patients may be salvaged.

COMMON ERRORS IN CARDIAC SCANNING

1. Neglecting to attempt the subcostal view in a person with an ectomorphic habitus
2. Failure to note diastolic collapse of the atria or ventricles when a pericardial effusion is noted
3. Failure to note marked hyper- or hypokinesis of the ventricles when an effusion is not present
4. Neglecting to note valve motion or wall motion when looking for electromechanical dissociation
5. Mistaking motion caused by positive-pressure ventilation for cardiac motion
6. Failure to note evidence of loculation when pericardial fluid is noted
7. Confusion of left- and right-sided heart chambers due to improper transducer orientation
8. Overdiagnosing pericardial effusion: confusion with pleural effusion or hypoechoic pericardial fat
9. Failure to position patient for optimal acoustic window

SELECTED READINGS

A complete bibliography pertaining to cardiac application is found on page 195.

CHAPTER 3

Other Emergency Department Applications

Abdominal Applications

APPENDICITIS

The most common emergency department diagnosis leading to urgent surgery is appendicitis. Much has been written in both the surgical and emergency medicine literature regarding the diagnosis of appendicitis, and virtually all of it emphasizes the importance of clinical history and examination above all else. Imaging procedures have traditionally had little to add to the diagnostic work-up, but use of the barium enema, particularly in children, has received some attention and continues to be used in some institutions. For the past decade, and particularly in the last 5 years, interest has developed in using ultrasound to aid in the diagnosis of the questionable case. Data from Europe (and more recently from the United States) seem to be very encouraging, with sensitivities of approximately 80 to 90% and specificities of 95% when graded compression techniques are used, but there is no doubt that the study is user dependent and requires considerable experience in order to perform it reliably. Although the role of ultrasound in the diagnosis of emergency appendicitis is undefined, its continued investigation and use by ultrasonographers is expanding

rapidly. It is clearly an area in which cooperation and ongoing communication between the emergency physician and the radiologists will prove beneficial to both.

Sonographic Considerations

Even with excellent instrumentation and experienced sonographers, the normal appendix is rarely visualized. This is not surprising, because appendix tissue is no different than that of the adjacent bowel. The appendix wall is normally less than or equal to 6 mm, and it compresses easily with transducer pressure. When acutely inflamed, these characteristics change and the structure becomes both larger and less compressible (Fig. 3–1). By very gradually increasing pressure with the transducer, the normal bowel and its contents are compressed. With experience, the area of the ileocecal junction can be identified and the iliac artery and vein and psoas muscle are identified as landmarks deep to the region of the appendix. Figure 3–2A and B illustrates the appearance of acute appendicitis. It consists of a noncompressible ring with a wall diameter equal to or greater than 7 mm. This structure should correspond to the point of

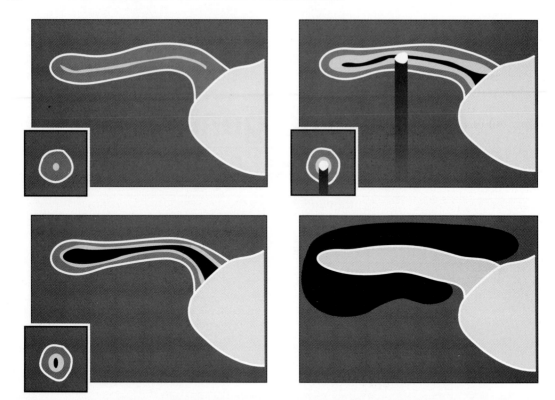

Figure 3-1. Acute appendicitis. Initially, the inflamed appendix appears dilated and noncompressible, without fluid in the lumen of the appendix (*top left*). Occasionally, an appendicolith is visualized within the lumen of the appendix (*top right*). In gangrenous appendicitis, the lumen of the appendix fills with fluid (*bottom left*). If the appendix has perforated, the appendix may be difficult to visualize; if seen, it appears as an echogenic projection surrounded by anechoic fluid (*bottom right*).

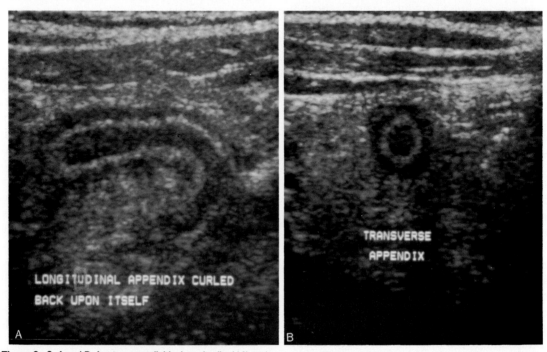

Figure 3-2. *A* and *B*, Acute appendicitis. Longitudinal (*A*) and transverse (*B*) views of a dilated, noncompressible appendix in a patient with appendicitis. The appendiceal diameter measures 9 mm in these images (≥7 mm and noncompressibility is strongly suggestive of acute appendicitis).

maximal tenderness, which at times is far from McBurney's point. In the patient with an appendicolith (concretion of fecal matter), this may be visualized within the appendix. Figure 3–3 illustrates this finding, which is much more common on ultrasound than on plain radiographs. All of the known complications of appendicitis, including gangrene, perforation, and phlegmon, have been described sonographically. In a female patient with right-sided abdominal pain and a negative ultrasound examination for appendicitis, pelvic ultrasound is usually the next step. In difficult cases of lower quadrant pain, it may be reasonable to refer the patient for ultrasound evaluation of the appendix and sonography of the kidney and gallbladder as well. This "pansonography" of the abdomen and pelvis is being used more often.

Clinical Considerations

The vast majority of emergency department patients with suspected appendicitis do not warrant ultrasound (unless it is being done in a conscious effort to give the sonographer experience!), plain radiographs of the abdomen, or any imaging technique, with the possible exception of a chest x-ray. In the questionable case, however, ultrasound has already proved to be a valuable adjunct in some institutions and well may become generally accepted as the prime diagnostic test in such cases as experience is accrued. In the borderline case, the benefits of ultrasound are already clear. In the patient in whom appendiceal perforation has already occurred and peritoneal signs are prominent, the examination is less useful. This is due to the difficulty in applying pressure because pain is solicited and to the distortion of anatomy that occurs in the inflamed appendiceal region. In such a situation, the examination is nondiagnostic for appendicitis, but often indicates abnormalities that warrant further investigation. It is important that the emergency physician who wishes to obtain ultrasound on patients with suspected appendicitis understands this seeming paradox: the technique is actually more useful (specific) in early stages of the disease. Recent reports of patients with rather typical clinical and ultrasound evidence of acute appendicitis (without mechanical obstruction of the appendix) who have resolved spontaneously may help provide new insight into the natural history of this common disease. Often, the greatest benefit of right lower quadrant scanning combined with transvaginal or transabdominal pelvic scanning is the identification of the cause of nonappendiceal pain.

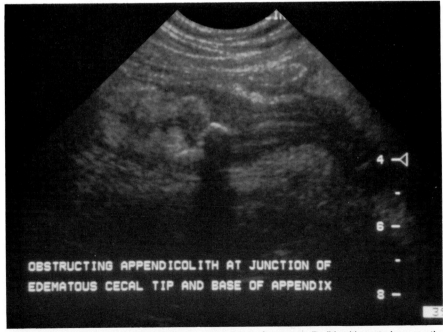

Figure 3–3. Appendicolith. This sonogram illustrates the appearance of an appendicolith with posterior acoustic shadowing. These occur in approximately 10 to 15% of cases of acute appendicitis and are associated with a high incidence of perforation.

SONOGRAPHY OF OTHER LOWER ABDOMINAL CONDITIONS

Several other conditions of interest to the emergency physician are largely an outgrowth of appendiceal scanning. Inflammation of the terminal ilium, either from Crohn's disease or infectious causes, may be demonstrated with ultrasound. Thickening and lack of compressibility of the bowel wall are the chief findings. In some cases, unnecessary laparotomy has been avoided. The much-invoked and previously little-proved diagnosis of mesenteric adenitis has also been identified by ultrasound. The enlarged mesenteric nodes appear as multiple hypoechoic structures. Diverticular disease of the colon is also an area of active ultrasound investigation. For uncomplicated diverticulitis, ultrasound examination is less likely to be useful than traditional contrast studies, although some changes, principally mural thickening, may be observed. For complications of diverticulitis, especially abscess and fistula formation, ultrasound may prove to be an effective and noninvasive way to confirm the diagnosis and assess the results of therapy. From the standpoint of an emergency physician, the formation of any extracolonic manifestation of diverticular disease mandates admission rather than out-patient therapy. Figure 3–4 shows normal bowel.

These ultrasound uses just discussed are somewhat novel, but are employed clinically on a regular basis in some centers. The only certainty is that the abdominal applications of ultrasound are relevant to the emergency physician and will continue to increase.

HEPATIC AND HEPATOBILIARY SCANNING

There are virtually no true emergency indications for hepatic scanning apart from those discussed in sections on trauma and the biliary tract. Obviously, patients with known hepatic or splenic disease ranging from hepatic abscess and Wilson's disease to Budd-Chiari syndrome appear in the emergency department. Ultrasound examinations are usually ordered in these patients for comparison with old studies, but true emergency applications of these scans are rare. The liver and spleen are easily visualized while performing other studies (in fact they are the two abdominal organs used most frequently as acoustic windows), and it is useful to know something of their ultrasound characteristics in common pathologic states.

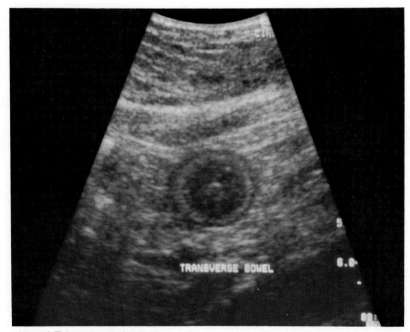

Figure 3–4. Normal bowel. This transverse image depicts the normal target appearance of bowel in cross section. If there is a sufficient amount of fluid in the lumen, motion of particulate matter can be observed in real-time scanning.

Sonographic Considerations

The ultrasound appearance of the liver soon becomes clear to anyone who performs abdominal ultrasound. Figures 1–26 and 1–27 demonstrate typical long-axis views in which the parenchyma is seen to be slightly more echogenic than the adjacent kidney. The major venous systems, including the hepatic veins, the portal veins, and the vena cava, constitute most of the branching tubular structures noted (Figs. 3–5 and 3–6); the normal bile ducts are not usually visualized peripherally within the liver. The diaphragm is visible in most liver scans (Fig. 3–7) and it appears brighter than liver parenchyma; this is due to the presence of a greater number of reflective surfaces in the diaphragm in comparison to the adjacent liver. The most common diseases that affect the liver—fatty infiltration (Fig. 3–8A) and cirrhosis (Fig. 3–8B–D)—cause a generalized increase in the echogenicity, although regenerating cirrhotic nodules may have an inhomogeneous appearance.

Acute hepatitis is described as having accentuated brightness of the walls of the portal veins, but these changes are too subtle to be relied on consistently in the emergency department. Liver size is often of clinical relevance and can be readily measured with bedside ultrasound. The greatest long axis as measured from the right diaphragm to the tip of the liver normally is less than 13.5 cm; anything over 15.5 cm suggests hepatomegaly. Few of the many possible focal lesions merit description here. Metastatic colon carcinoma (Fig. 3–9A–C) and hemangiomas (Fig. 3–10A and B) generally appear as echogenic nodules. Other metastatic diseases and hepatocellular carcinoma have a more variable ultrasound appearance (hypoechoic, isoechoic, hyperechoic, inhomogeneous, target, etc.). Cystic lesions look exactly like what would be predicted, with an anechoic center surrounded by a thin wall (Fig. 3–11). Hepatic abscesses appear (as do abscesses elsewhere) as more complex combinations of low echogenicity (Fig. 3–12A and B). The emergency physician is not expected to precisely diagnose these and all other focal hepatic diseases (Fig. 3–12C–E). In most cases, however, recognition of the abnormal appearance of focal hepatic disease is possible and an appropriate diagnostic work-up is initiated.

Hepatobiliary Tree

It might at first seem paradoxical that ultrasound evaluation of the hepatobiliary tree, primarily identification of the intra- and extrahepatic biliary ducts, should be distinct from gallbladder scanning itself. It makes sense,

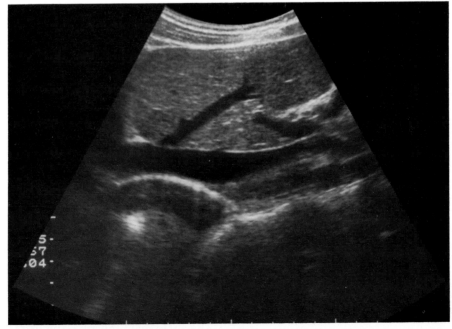

Figure 3–5. Longitudinal scan of normal liver. Hepatic veins appear as thin-walled structures and can be seen entering the inferior vena cava (immediately below the liver).

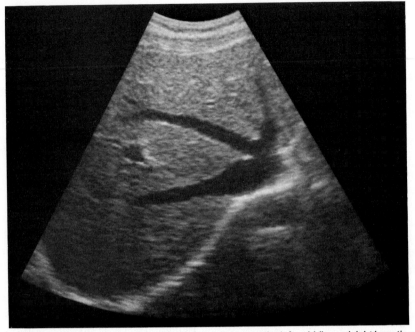

Figure 3–6. Hepatic venous anatomy. This transverse view demonstrates the left, middle, and right hepatic veins merging as they enter the inferior vena cava.

however, because despite the fact that the gallbladder and biliary tree are closely related (both anatomically and functionally), the ultrasound evaluation is very different and the clinical indications for the studies are quite distinct as well. Although scanning of the gallbladder is quite straightforward and pathology of the gallblad-

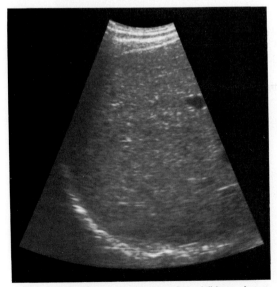

Figure 3–7. Diaphragm. The diaphragm is visible as a hyperechoic structure in the left lower portion of the image.

der is usually easily recognized, the evaluation of the hepatobiliary tree is much more subtle and complex and abnormalities are much less likely to be found in the typical emergency department population. Although it is clearly useful and perhaps necessary for the emergency physician to understand the role of ultrasound, particularly in the evaluation of jaundice, the actual delineation of ductal abnormalities is neither consistently feasible nor vital to the emergency practitioner. The goals of the emergency practitioner, therefore, should be to know when ultrasound evaluation of the tree is indicated in the emergency department patient and what the advantages and limitations of ultrasound are in this evaluation. Most commonly, the emergency physician is called on to recognize what the diagnostic and therapeutic implications are when actual dilatation is found either during the course of a gallbladder scan or as a result of a formal hepatobiliary ultrasound, nuclear medicine scan, or computed tomography (CT) examination.

Sonographic Considerations of the Hepatobiliary Tree

The anatomy of the intra-and extrahepatic bile ducts and their closely associated vascular

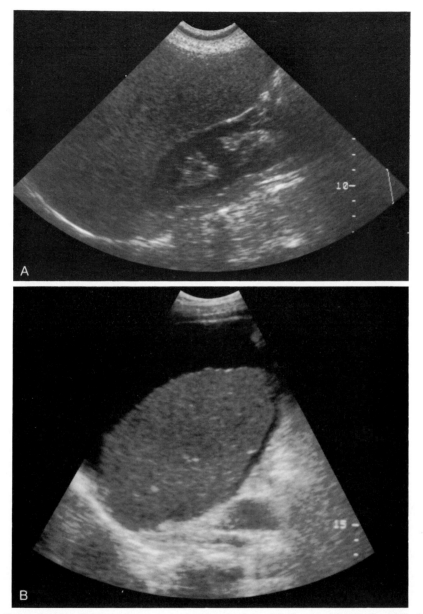

Figure 3-8. *A*, Fatty infiltration. The liver demonstrates increased echogenicity in comparison to the relatively hyperechoic renal cortex. In addition, there is impaired visualization of the intrahepatic vessels and diaphragm, suggesting a moderate to severe degree of fatty infiltration. *B–D*, Cirrhosis. The shrunken liver demonstrates increased echogenicity and a nodular border. There is a large amount of ascitic fluid surrounding the liver and gallbladder. The ascitic fluid conveys the appearance of gallbladder wall thickening, seen in *D*.

structures is complex. The simplified view shown in Figure 2–2 is complicated enough but gives little appreciation of the difficulties associated with proper ultrasound identification of these structures. In many regions, the structures are superimposed and intertwined. Even under normal conditions, the distinction between arteries, veins, and biliary ducts is not always ob-

vious. Moreover, the extrahepatic biliary tree can be difficult to visualize due to artifact created by interposed loops of bowel. Finally, it is frequently necessary to use multiple different and nonstandard acoustic windows in order to visualize these structures; thus, imaging the hepatobiliary tree mandates a profound understanding of normal and abnormal anatomy, as

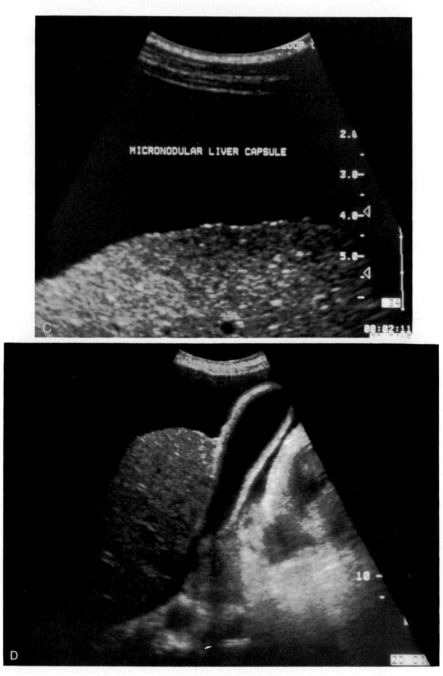

Figure 3-8 *Continued*

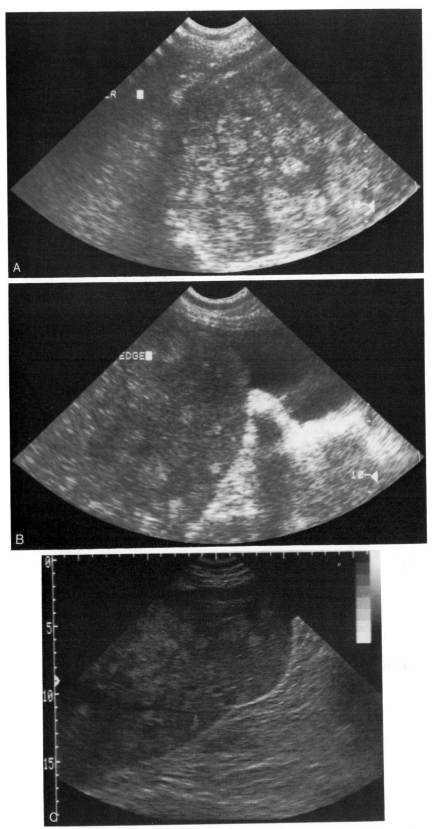

Figure 3-9. *A–C*, Metastatic colon carcinoma. Metastatic disease to the liver is more common than primary hepatic carcinoma. These images demonstrate multiple echogenic foci within the liver. Cancer of the colon is the tumor that is most frequently associated with this appearance.

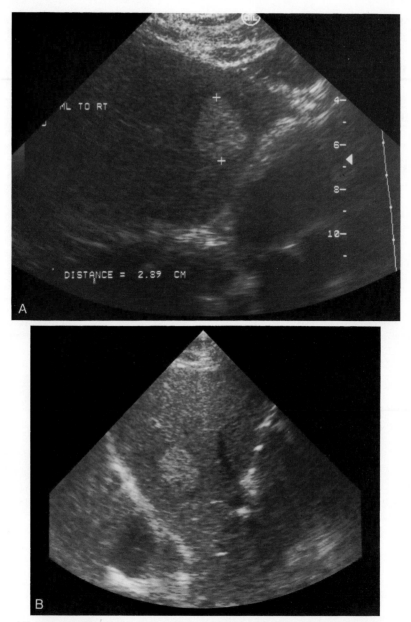

Figure 3–10. A and B, Hemangiomas. This homogeneous, well-marginated, echodense appearance is typical for hemangiomas. This is the most common benign tumor of the liver. Approximately three quarters of hemangiomas are found in the right lobe of the liver and are seen more frequently in women and the elderly.

well as considerable experience in performing ultrasound. Radiologists are wont to say that ultrasound is the most difficult of all imaging studies. This oversimplification finds its just application in sonography of the hepatobiliary tree.

It is conceptually clear that the great importance of identification of dilated bile ducts is the implication that an obstructing lesion is present.

If jaundice was the indication for obtaining the ultrasound examination, the presence of biliary obstruction excludes hepatocellular disease from the differential diagnosis. One limitation to remember is that it appears to take approximately 48 hours for dilatation of the biliary tract to begin after the onset of total obstruction. Furthermore, the extrahepatic portion seems to dilate more readily than the intrahepatic portions.

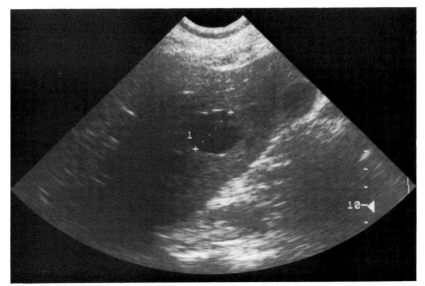

Figure 3–11. Hepatic cysts. Cysts in the liver are relatively common in the elderly. They may be congenital, inflammatory, parasitic, traumatic, or of unknown cause. Hepatic cysts should be anechoic, with well-defined walls and posterior acoustic enhancement. These cysts occasionally may contain slender septa. The characteristic appearance of typical hepatic cysts usually requires no further work-up. If the diagnosis is in question, ultrasound-guided aspiration may be of diagnostic value.

Despite this, it is dilatation of intrahepatic bile ducts that is most likely to be noted as an incidental finding in gallbladder or general abdominal scanning; this is because normal intrahepatic bile ducts are not ordinarily visualized in ultrasound of the liver. When dilated, however, intrahepatic bile ducts may become quite prominent and are an almost infallible indicator of obstruction (Fig. 3–13A and B). Although local disease of the liver can cause intrahepatic dilatation, it is far more common that obstruction occurs in the relatively small extrahepatic duct system. There is some evidence that dilatation of the extrahepatic bile ducts may be noted even before the onset of clinical jaundice. The goal of hepatobiliary scanning is to examine the extrahepatic ducts in order to establish the level at which the obstruction has occurred, if not the cause of the obstructive process. Both the common hepatic and common bile ducts are usually visualized with standard ultrasound equipment. Figure 3–14 shows the typical appearance of the common hepatic duct with its thick wall and small internal diameter (normally less than 4 mm). The precise junction of the common hepatic duct and common bile duct is often not well visualized (Fig. 3–15), and the sonographically identified structure is referred to simply as the common duct. Normal values for the common bile duct's internal diameter range up to 7 mm; dilatation of the common bile duct is illustrated in Figure 3–16. Stones impacted in the extrahepatic biliary duct may or may not be visualized with ultrasound (Fig. 3–17A and B); in many cases, endoscopic retrograde cholangiopancreatography (ERCP) is required. An infected and obstructed biliary tree constitutes an acute surgical emergency. The clinical presentation of acute cholangitis mandates documentation or refutation of biliary obstruction. Ultrasound, CT, ERCP, and transhepatic cholangiography are all appropriate options. It should be remembered that stones can form in the bile ducts themselves, even in the absence of a gallbladder; this is called primary choledocholithiasis.

Clinical Considerations

The emergency physician may encounter dilated bile ducts as an incidental finding during gallbladder ultrasound. In such cases, this finding may be truly incidental, unrelated to gallbladder disease, or may be the result of a proximally impacted stone. At times, the underlying diagnosis is immediately obvious (e.g., "there is a large mass seen in the head of the pancreas with evidence of multiple metastatic lesions in

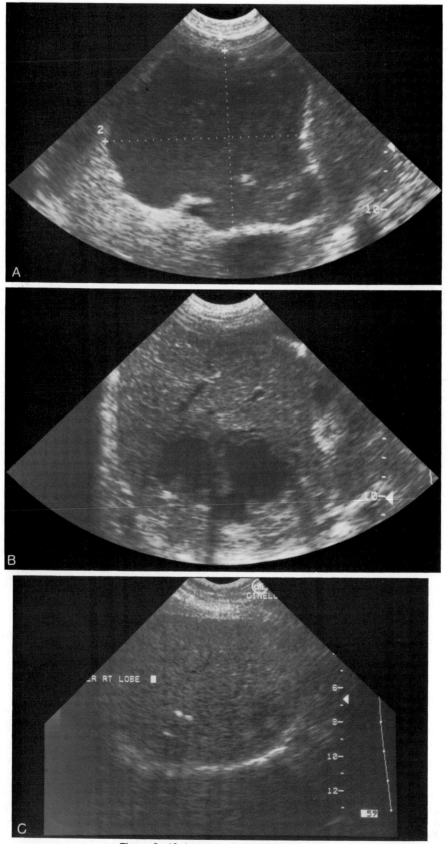

Figure 3–12. *Legend on opposite page.*

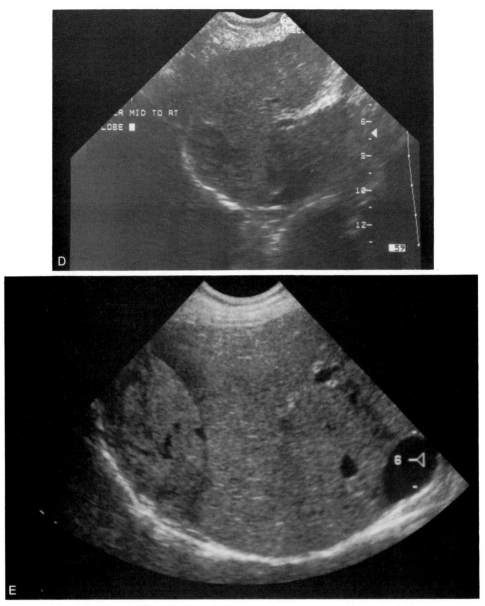

Figure 3-12. *A* and *B*, Hepatic abscess. These images demonstrate the appearance of a hepatic abscess prior to (*A*) and following (*B*) percutaneous drainage of 600 mL of purulent material. On ultrasound examination, these abscesses usually have irregular, thick walls and a hypoechoic central area that may contain some debris. Abscesses may be bacterial (*Escherichia coli* and anaerobic), amebic parasitic, or fungal in cause. *C*, Hepatic calcifications. Bacterial infections, parasitic disease, trauma, syphilis, tuberculosis, and other chronic granulomatous diseases have been associated with echogenic foci in the liver. *D*, Hypoechoic complex liver mass. This appearance can be seen with primary hepatic tumors, metastatic disease, older hematomas, and infectious processes. *E*, Hepatic hematoma. The hematoma in this image is subcapsular and of (isoechoic) similar echogenicity to the neighboring liver parenchyma. Trauma is the leading cause of hepatic hematomas, although they occasionally may be associated with spontaneous rupture of a hemangioma, tumor, or pseudoaneurysm. Very early on, acute bleeding may appear hypoechoic. The hematoma subsequently appears echogenic as a result of clot formation and fibrin deposition. With time, this area usually appears progressively less echogenic; however, liver hematomas have a variable appearance, depending on the age, organization, scarring, and calcification of the hematoma.

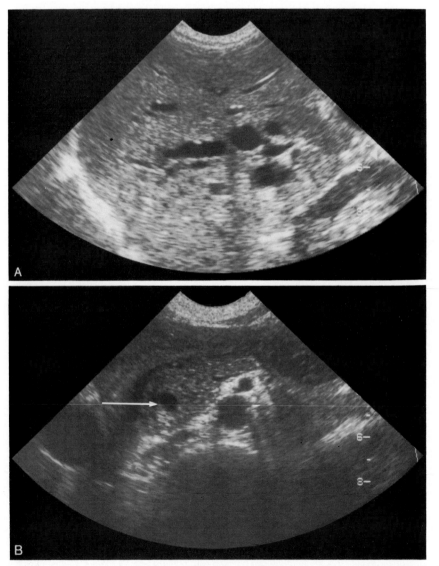

Figure 3–13. *A* and *B*, Dilated intrahepatic bile ducts. *A*, The ultrasound appearance of dilated intrahepatic bile ducts. *B*, A transverse image at the level of pancreas that illustrates dilatation of the intrapancreatic common bile duct (*arrow*) in a patient with pancreatic carcinoma. Dilatation of the extrahepatic biliary system occurs within 24 hours of acute obstruction, whereas dilatation of the intrahepatic ducts usually occurs several days later. The presence of dilated intrahepatic bile ducts is specific for biliary obstruction; however, it is not very sensitive, because approximately one quarter of patients with obstruction have normal size intrahepatic ducts.

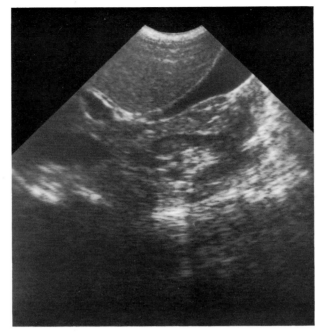

Figure 3-14. Normal common hepatic duct. The common hepatic duct is visualized anterior to the right portal vein and measures less than 4 mm.

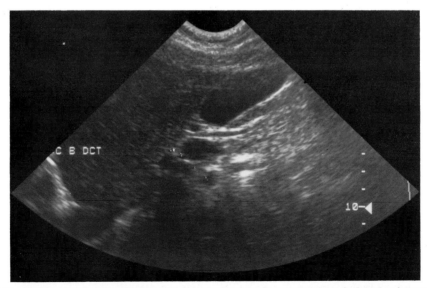

Figure 3-15. Common duct. Often the insertion of the cystic duct into the common hepatic duct that forms the bile duct is poorly visualized. Some authors use the phrase "common duct" to describe the junction of the common hepatic duct with the bile duct in this setting.

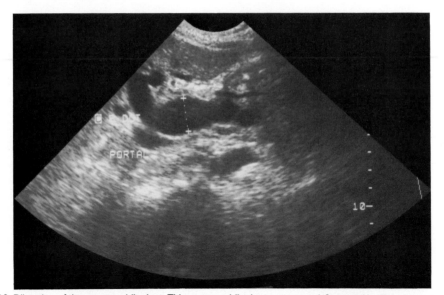

Figure 3–16. Dilatation of the common bile duct. This common bile duct measures 1.9 cm and is dilated as a result of a carcinoma at the head of the pancreas.

the liver"); at times, the diagnosis is obscure, but documentation of dilated bile ducts virtually always has profound implications in terms of admission and referral. The emergency department work-up of hepatocellular versus obstructive jaundice might reasonably include bedside scanning. The presence of dilated intrahepatic ducts would immediately mandate an inpatient work-up to define and alleviate the obstructing process.

SPLEEN

The spleen is most commonly visualized in the emergency department setting when it is used as an acoustic window for scanning the left kidney. In adults, it characteristically has a crescent shape when viewed in sagittal section and appears as a homogeneous structure of medium echogenicity, with the hyperechoic left diaphragm forming the posterior border, as seen in Figure 3–18.

Bedside ultrasound may be useful for confirming suspected splenic enlargement but, due to its rather variable shape, no single measurement reliably distinguishes normal from abnormal. As a general guide, on transverse supine scan the anteroposterior diameter should be at least twice the width, and the most caudad portion should not extend significantly below the left costal margin. Moderate enlargement is usually quite evident (Fig. 3–19A–C), particularly when splenic size is compared to that of the liver.

Both the stomach and the lung may interfere with splenic visualization; placing the patient in a slight or moderate right-side-down decubitus position is often helpful.

Although splenic lacerations may be visualized with ultrasound (Fig. 3–20A–C), it is clear that CT is a far more sensitive technique. Splenic hematomas, cysts, and infarctions are all recognized by their abnormal ultrasound characteristics against the homogeneous background of normal splenic parenchyma. An older splenic hematoma is demonstrated in Figure 3–21A and B.

STOMACH

The stomach would appear to be a poor candidate for ultrasonic visualization, particularly in view of the much better radiographic and endoscopic techniques that are available. After distention with water, the stomach has been used as an acoustic window to visualize the pancreas and surrounding structures; some descriptions of the ultrasound appearance of gastric contents have appeared.

It has been suggested that ultrasound should be used as an emergency procedure to confirm

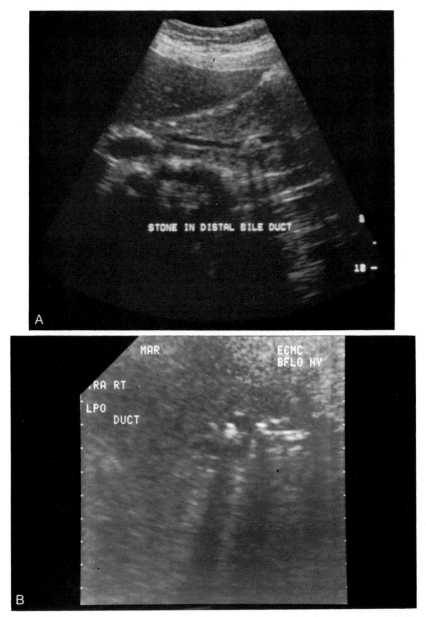

Figure 3–17. A and B, Stones in common bile duct. Choledocholithiasis is demonstrated by the presence of echogenic material within the common bile duct. The stones are less likely to cause posterior acoustic shadowing because of their smaller size. The proximal common bile duct can usually be identified; however, the distal portion of the duct is very difficult to see because of overlying bowel gas. As a result, a large number of common bile duct stones are missed on ultrasound examination.

the ingestion of pills in the patient who presents with suspected or known overdose. It is already clear that only sustained-release preparations are even theoretically visible for a significant time, and much more data are needed before it is established what, if any role, ultrasound would add to the management of the poisoned patient. It seems more logical, although it has

not been demonstrated, that ultrasound could play a role in the detection of gastric bezoars.

A new use of gastric ultrasound is to confirm the presence of food in the stomach. This was studied in order to identify patients at risk for aspiration during childbirth, but it may have application in the emergency department setting. Although the empty stomach is not visual-

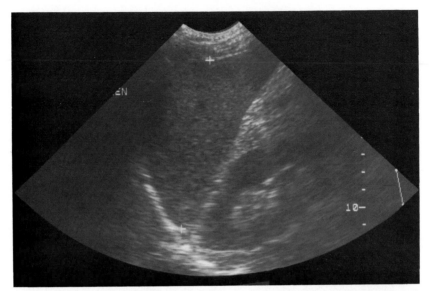

Figure 3–18. Normal spleen. The spleen is identified between the two markers in this image. The diaphragm is to the left of the spleen, and the kidney is identified to its right.

ized, the ingestion of 2 cups of water reliably allows the identification of food in the stomach. Using the 5-MHz transducer and a sitting posture, investigators confirmed the absence of food in all normal fasting volunteers and the presence of food in all volunteers after a standard meal. Repeat scanning documented an absence of food in all normal subjects by 4 hours postprandially. Although the clinical emphasis of the study was on identifying patients in active labor at risk for aspiration (and greatly delayed gastric emptying was noted in this population), potential emergency department application as a means of identifying patients in need of gastric emptying is apparent. It is notable that identification of the stomach was confirmed by observing the entry of ingested water into the stomach on real-time ultrasound. Figure 3–22 demonstrates the appearance of a fluid-filled stomach, pylorus, and duodenum.

PANCREAS

Ultrasound examination of the pancreas often is not easy to either perform or interpret, nor is it particularly sensitive or specific. In cases of mild acute pancreatitis, normal findings are common. However, instances where the pancreas is noted to be enlarged and the internal echogenicity is decreased are strong confirmatory evidence of acute pancreatitis. It is conceivable that these findings might be seen on abdominal ultrasound examination in a patient with obscure abdominal pain. In patients with chronic pancreatitis, commonly described sonographic findings include an atrophied gland, localized areas of enlargement, increased echogenicity, and dilatation of the main pancreatic duct. The fact that sonography of the pancreas is often normal in the patient who has been labeled with chronic pancreatitis may be due to either the relative insensitivity of the sonographic diagnosis or to the uncertainty of the clinical diagnosis. Examination of the emergency department patient with known or suspected pseudocysts, however, is far more rewarding. The normal anatomy of this region is interesting and complex and mandates some study for proper interpretation. Figures 3–23 and 3–24 show transverse scanning at the epigastrium; the body of the pancreas, the inferior vena cava, the aorta, the splenic vein, the superior mesenteric artery, and the liver are all visualized. Examples of chronic pancreatitis, dilated pancreatic ducts, and a pancreatic pseudocyst are illustrated in Figures 3–25 to 3–27.

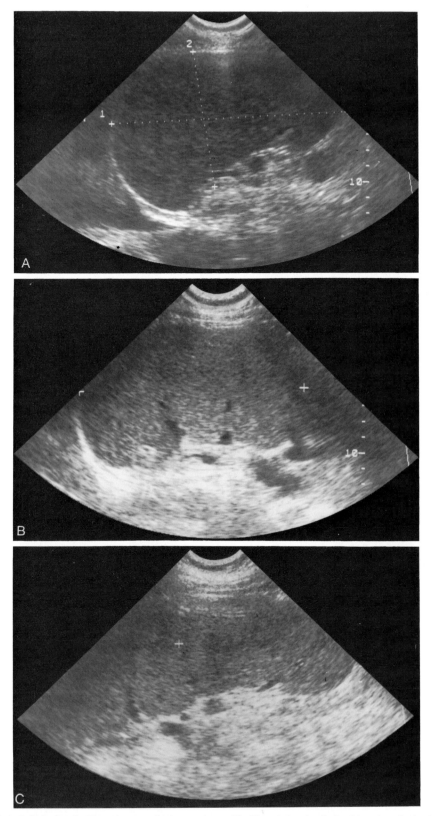

Figure 3–19. A, Splenomegaly. These images display moderate (A, 15 cm in longitudinal axis) and marked splenomegaly (B and C, 26 cm in longitudinal axis).

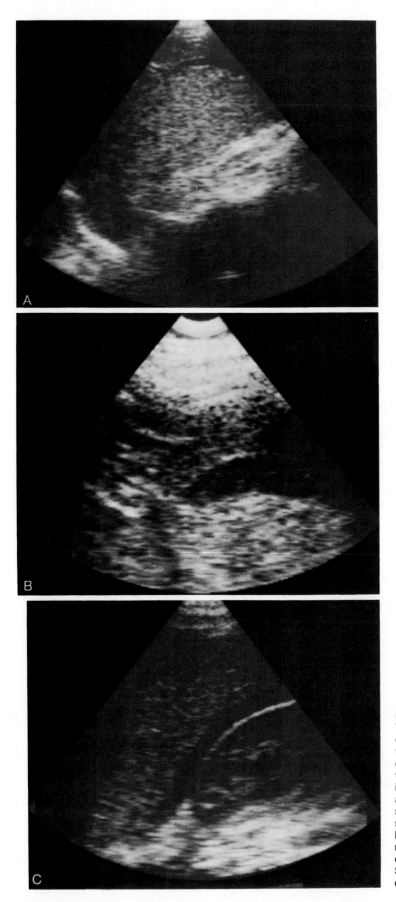

Figure 3–20. *A–C.* Splenic rupture. This patient with mononucleosis developed a splenic tear with no significant trauma. The splenic laceration is apparent in the uppermost portion of *A* and in the central portion of the magnified image in *B*. It appears as an anechoic area within the spleen. Imaging of Morison's pouching reveals an anechoic stripe as a result of the intraperitoneal hemorrhage. Mononucleosis is the most common cause of "spontaneous" splenic rupture in the United States, whereas malaria is the most common etiologic factor worldwide.

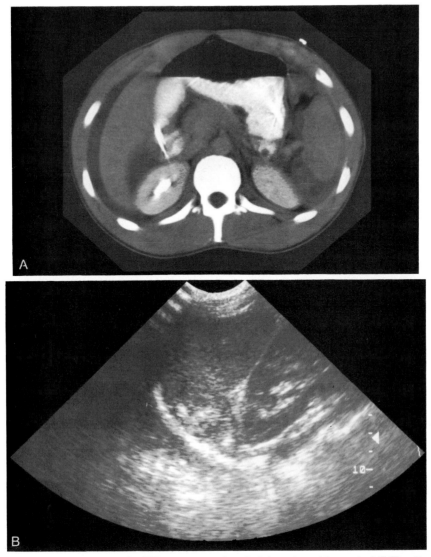

Figure 3–21. *A,* The computed tomography (CT) appearance of a splenic hematoma (plus marker). *B,* The ultrasound appearance of this splenic hematoma months later. There are areas of increased echogenicity (scar or calcification) corresponding with the location of the hematoma on the CT scan.

INTRAPERITONEAL FLUID (ASCITES)

The identification of nontraumatic peritoneal fluid is quite important in emergency medicine. Most commonly, the ascitic fluid is the result of cirrhosis, congestive heart failure, or hypoalbuminemia. In such cases, the onset of ascites may well indicate a deterioration in the underlying condition. Often, admission or at least a change in therapy is indicated. Other sources of intraperitoneal fluid may be chylous ascites, which indicates disruption of thoracic lymphatic duct or other elements of the lymphatic duct system; this is characterized by its milky appearance. Perforation of viscera can result in small or moderate amounts of intraperitoneal fluid, and intraabdominal abscesses often produce small collections of fluid that may be free or loculated in the affected area (e.g., the pericolic region). In such cases, the discovery of intraperitoneal fluids is a clue that leads directly to the diagnosis of the underlying disease.

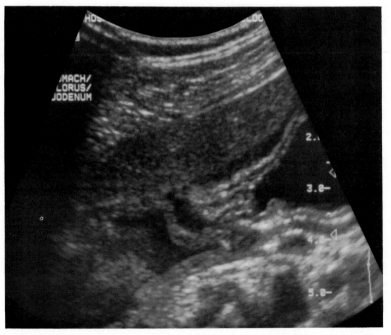

Figure 3–22. Normal stomach pylorus and duodenum. When these structures are fluid filled, they may be visualized well with ultrasound.

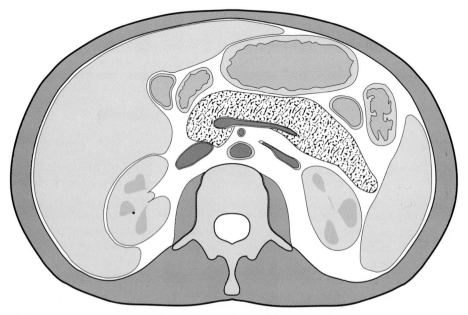

Figure 3–23. Pancreas. The appearance of the pancreas and surrounding organs in a transverse section of the upper abdomen. The splenic vein runs parallel to the pancreas, whereas the superior mesenteric artery and aorta are seen perpendicular to the pancreas.

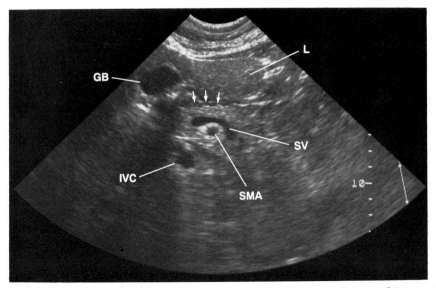

Figure 3–24. Normal pancreas. The upper border of the pancreas is outlined by the small arrows. Other structures that are well visualized in this image include liver (L), splenic vein (SV), superior mesenteric artery (SMA), inferior vena cava (IVC), and gallbladder (GB).

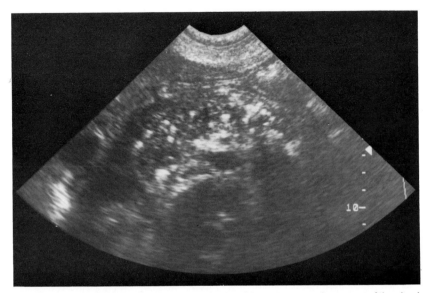

Figure 3–25. Chronic pancreatitis. There is increased echogenicity of the pancreas, enlargement of the gland, and irregularity of the outline of the pancreas typically seen with chronic pancreatitis. There are multiple pancreatic calcifications with posterior shadowing that give the gland a stippled appearance.

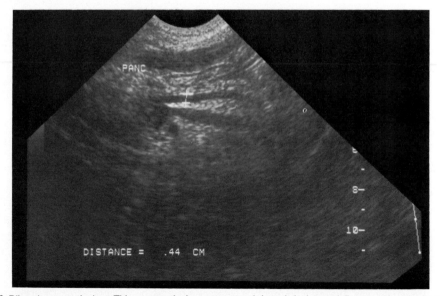

Figure 3–26. Dilated pancreatic duct. This pancreatic duct measures 4.4 mm in its internal diameter. A normal pancreatic duct measures ≤2 mm. Dilatation is frequently seen in association with chronic pancreatitis and has been reported to be present in over 90% of patients who demonstrate pancreatic calcifications.

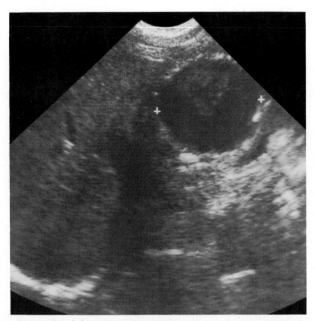

Figure 3–27. Pancreatic pseudocyst. This 6.6-cm diameter cystic structure has sharply defined walls and demonstrates posterior acoustic enhancement. There are some internal echoes within the cyst. The majority of pseudocysts are associated with pancreatitis; most of the remaining cases are secondary to direct trauma. Pseudocysts are usually single and may result in dilatation of the pancreatic duct.

Sonographic Considerations

Ultrasound has been shown to be a sensitive method for detecting fluid in the peritoneal cavity. By some accounts, as little as 2 teaspoons of fluid is visualizable in the carefully performed examination, although this seems unrealistic (and recent studies during lavage indicate that perhaps 250 to 500 mL is needed to ensure visualization). Bland ascites is essentially a transudate believed to weep directly from the liver surface into the peritoneal cavity. When it appears during ultrasound examination as a dark, nonreflective layer between two rather reflective surfaces, it is readily identified. Other fluids, which often contain blood clots (e.g., malignant ascites), are characterized by some degree of echogenicity, particularly in the most dependent portion of the fluid collection. Large quantities of free-flowing ascites change the ultrasound appearance of the abdomen. Figures 3–28 and 3–29 indicate how ascites surrounds loops of small bowel and mesentery. Because the ascites acts as a perfect acoustic window, excellent detail (Fig. 3–30) is noted and certain structures that are not ordinarily well visualized are shown to advantage. The emergency department physician may wish to scan patients with ascites precisely for this reason.

When looking for possible intraperitoneal fluid, there are at least three areas where scanning proves rewarding. Extrapolating from studies done in the trauma setting (which may not be totally applicable), all three areas must be investigated for maximum sensitivity. One is the cul-de-sac (the pouch of Douglas), where ultrasound may normally demonstrate a very small amount of fluid during early pregnancy or after ovulation. Transvaginal ultrasound should be an extremely sensitive technique for this region. The space between the liver and the kidney (where Glisson's capsule adjoins Gerota's fascia) is also an excellent location for the visualization of small quantities of fluid (Fig. 3–31). The region between the spleen and left kidney is another area where free fluid is often identified. All these locations are helpful for the identification of fluid because of their relatively dependent positions and their rather hyperechoic surfaces, which contrast strikingly with the anechoic fluid.

Clinical Considerations

Physical examination and plain radiographs are notoriously inaccurate for the detection of ascites. The classic x-ray findings of "ground-glass" appearance, mid-line location of floating loops of bowel, and widening of the peritoneal fat stripe are insensitive (requiring many hundreds of milliliters of fluid) and often misleading. This is even more true for the classic physical examination findings of shifting dullness and fluid wave, which can be particularly

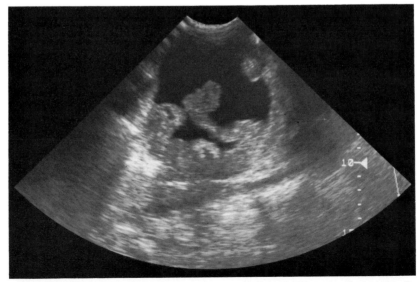

Figure 3–28. Bowel and mesentery. This image demonstrates the appearance of bowel and mesentery floating in a large amount of ascitic fluid. The bowel is anchored posteriorly by the mesentery.

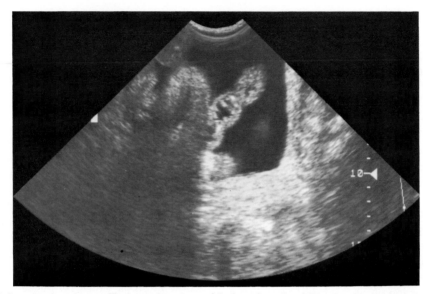

Figure 3–29. Bowel and mesentery. The internal structure of the bowel may be visible when it is floating in a large amount of ascitic fluid.

difficult to appreciate or falsely positive in obese patients. Bedside ultrasound examination, when used as an extension of physical diagnosis, enhances the physician's ability to identify peritoneal fluids with an accuracy approximate to CT examination. In those cases where laboratory examination of the fluid is required, such as Gram's stain and culture to rule out bacterial peritonitis, ultrasound is helpful in at least two ways: (1) it allows for aspiration of even small collections, which would be difficult to obtain if done blindly; and (2) it helps the physician to perform aspiration by identifying a route that avoids intraabdominal structures.

PLEURAL EFFUSION

Pleural effusions are included in the abdominal section of this text because the sonographic recognition is through abdominal scanning. Ultra-

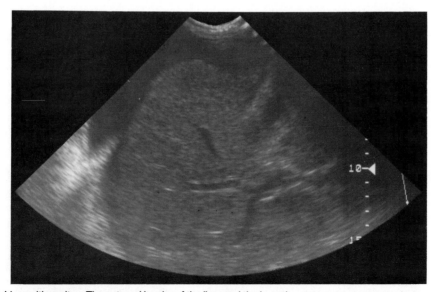

Figure 3–30. Liver with ascites. The external border of the liver and the hepatic venous structures are nicely seen in this patient who has a large amount of ascites.

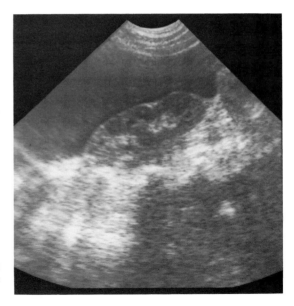

Figure 3–31. Fluid in Morison's pouch. The collection of fluid is visualized in the space between the liver and the right kidney.

sound is not usually thought of (particularly in the emergency department) as a primary means of making a diagnosis of pleural effusion, although it is capable of detecting small quantities of subpulmonic effusion that might not be seen on chest x-ray. Although certainly not a primary indication, it is important for the emergency physician to be able to recognize the appearance of pleural effusion, because it may have clinical importance when found on other scans.

The typical appearance of a pleural effusion is noted in Figures 3–32 to 3–34 and illustrated in Figure 3–35. Pleural effusion, or hemothorax for that matter, appears as an echo-free space distal to the hyperechoic line that represents the diaphragm. The liver acts as an excellent acous-

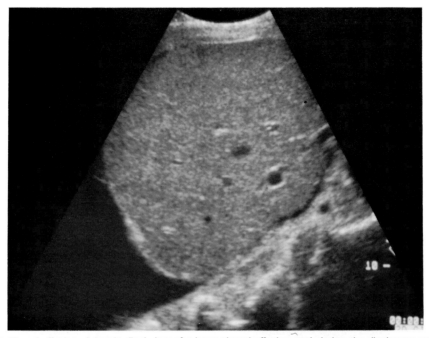

Figure 3–32. Pleural effusion. A longitudinal view of a large pleural effusion cephalad to the diaphragm and the liver.

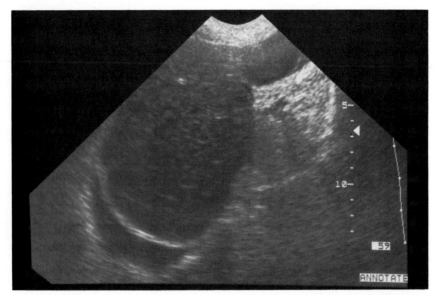

Figure 3-33. Pleural effusion. A transverse image of a pleural effusion posterior to the diaphragm and the liver.

tic window proximally, and the lower lung margin may be discernible. A similar appearance would be expected using the spleen as an acoustic window, but this region is less commonly scanned in the emergency department. The sonographic appearance of subdiaphragmatic fluid (Fig. 3-36) should not be confused with that of pleural fluid.

RENAL

There are occasional specialized cases other than acute obstructive uropathy where the emergency physician might well use renal ultrasound. The frequency varies greatly according to the facility, and such cases are ordinarily studied in the radiology suite by traditional ultrasound specialists using the highest quality equipment. It should be noted that renal vascular disorders, renal vein thrombosis, and acute renal infarction require Doppler ultrasound for investigation.

Renal transplant patients are a rapidly growing group who present frequently with renal problems. The specter of both infection and rejection is ever present, and these patients in-

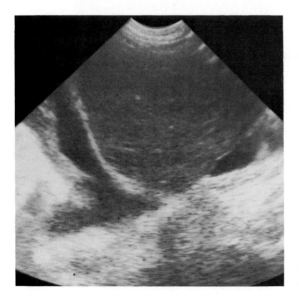

Figure 3-34. Pleural effusion. A smaller pleural effusion is visualized on the longitudinal scan.

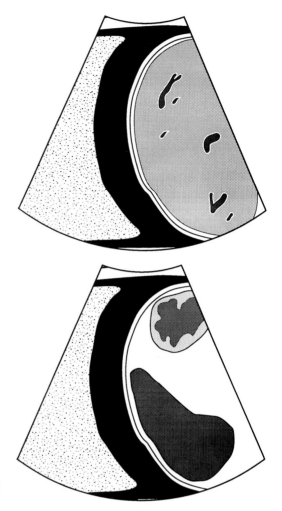

Figure 3–35. Pleural effusions. The ultrasound appearance of a right pleural effusion (*upper*) and left pleural effusion (*lower*).

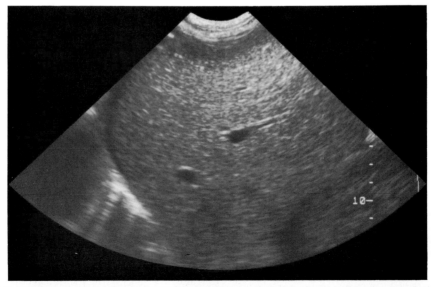

Figure 3–36. Subdiaphragmatic fluid. This image demonstrates an anechoic stripe between the echogenic diaphragm and the liver, which represents intraperitoneal fluid.

variably have some underlying renal disease; thus, contrast studies should be avoided. Several centers have developed special expertise in the ultrasound scanning of the transplanted renal patient. It is enough for the emergency physician to be aware that ultrasound plays a very prominent role in their evaluation. Transplanted kidneys have much the same appearance as natural organs, both normally and when diseased. Figures 2–58 and 3–37 illustrate the appearance of transplanted kidneys in the pelvis.

Trauma/Hematuria

The general question of ultrasound in the blunt trauma patient is dealt with in Chapter 2, "Hemoperitoneum." The specific condition of microscopic hematuria following rather mild trauma is a fairly common problem seen by the emergency physician. In many institutions, no imaging procedure is done and these patients are simply followed on an outpatient basis to see if their hematuria clears within several days to a week; if it does not, intravenous pyelography (IVP) is generally performed. It is possible to use bedside ultrasound during the first emergency department visit in order to screen for significant renal hematomas or renal fracture. This approach is particularly useful in those cases where the likelihood of follow-up and repeat urinalysis is uncertain.

Abdominal Masses

At times, a mass is palpated in the abdomen during a routine examination for abdominal or flank pain, but it is uncertain whether this represents an ectopic kidney or some other structure. Emergency department ultrasound will resolve the issue in identifying masses as ectopic kidney, renal cyst, or some other structure that requires further definition. Figure 3–38 shows a large renal cyst.

BLADDER

Although the urinary bladder is routinely used as an acoustic window to image the pelvic structures during transabdominal pelvic ultrasound, investigation of the bladder itself in the emergency department is limited to the quantification of residual urine.

It is often necessary in emergency department practice to determine whether a patient is able to empty his or her bladder completely. This most commonly occurs in the setting of elderly men who present with urinary frequency and in whom bladder neck obstruction is suspected. Occasionally, younger men with prostatitis present similarly. In these cases, an early step is to determine whether or not there is in fact urine in the bladder after voiding. The traditional method of doing this is straight or Foley catheterization, both of which carry a very real

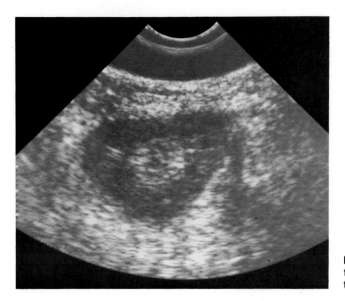

Figure 3–37. Transplanted kidney. This illustrates the appearance of a transplanted kidney on transverse view within the pelvis.

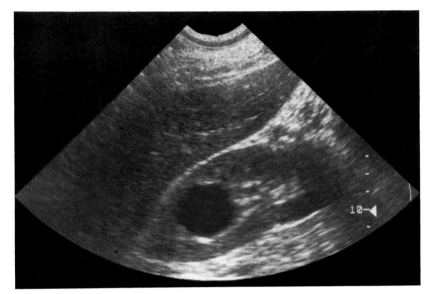

Figure 3-38. Large renal cyst. Most renal cysts arise from the parenchymal tissue, but occasionally cysts arise in the hilum. This cyst does not communicate with the collecting system and should not be confused with hydronephrosis.

risk of infection and can cause patient discomfort. In a great many cases, bedside ultrasound in the emergency department can replace this invasive procedure. As would be expected on the basis of physical properties, urine in the bladder is very easily visualized by sonography. Measurement of the bladder size can give a very accurate estimate of how much urine is present. For most purposes, it is sufficient to document whether the bladder is virtually empty after voiding or whether several hundred milliliters remain. Bladder volume (in milliliters) can be roughly calculated by the formula: transverse diameter multiplied by anteroposterior diameter multiplied by length (in centimeters) (others calculate bladder volume by assuming the bladder to be a sphere). In a similar manner, bedside ultrasound can be used to determine the status of the patient's bladder prior to transabdominal pelvic ultrasound. Patient preparation can then be directed accordingly. Conversely, bedside ultrasound can ensure an empty bladder prior to paracentesis or peritoneal lavage.

SELECTED READINGS

Abdominal Applications

Abu-Yousef MM, Franken EA: An overview of graded compression sonography in the diagnosis of acute appendicitis. Semin Ultrasound CT MR 1989;10:352.

Cooperberg P, Golding RH: Advances in ultrasonography of the gallbladder and biliary tract. Radiol Clin North Am 1982;20:611-633.

Crady SK, Jones JS, Wyn T, Luttenton CR: Clinical validity of US in children with suspected appendicitis. Ann Emerg Med 1993;22:1125-1129.

Forsby J, Henriksson L: Detectability of intraperitoneal fluid by ultrasonography. Acta Radiol Diagn 1984;25:375.

Heller MB, Skolnick ML: Ultrasound documentation of spontaneously resolving appendicitis. Am J Emerg Med 1993;11:51-53.

Hessel S, Siegelman S, McNeil B, et al: Prospective evaluation of computed tomography and ultrasound of the pancreas. Radiology 1982;143:129.

Lain FC, Jeffrey RB, Wing VW, Nyberg DA: Biliary dilatation: Defining the level and cause of real-time US. Radiology 1986;160:39-42.

Meyer MA: The spread and localization of acute peritoneal effusions. Radiology 1970;95:547-554.

Platt JF, Rubin JM, Ellis JH, et al: Duplex Doppler ultrasound of the kidney: Differentiation of obstructive from nonobstructive dilatation. Radiology 1989;171:515-517.

Puylaert JBC: Acute appendicitis: US evaluation using graded compression. Radiology 1986;158:355.

Siegel MJ, Carel C, Surratt S: Ultrasonography of acute abdominal pain in children. JAMA 1991;266:1987-1989.

Texts

For most other emergency department abdominal applications, the general abdominal texts noted in Chapter 2 are useful and a source for further references.

Goldberg B: Textbook of Abdominal Ultrasound. Baltimore: Williams & Wilkins, 1993. *Exceptional discussion and illustration of intraabdominal and pleural fluids. Many splenic images. Detailed discussion of bile duct obstruction.*

Jeffrey RB: CT and Sonography for the Acute Abdomen. New York: Raven Press, 1989. *Particularly good for demonstration of appendicitis and other inflammatory conditions.*

Gynecologic Applications

The primary use of emergency pelvic ultrasound in diagnosing and ruling out suspected ectopic pregnancy is fully discussed in Chapter 2. There are many other possible uses of pelvic ultrasound in the emergency department that are not necessarily related to problems of early pregnancy. In fact, the nature of the conditions involved and the characteristics of the pelvic anatomy often make pelvic sonography the procedure of choice in diagnosing a wide variety of diseases. The multiplicity of disease states and the variability of their ultrasound appearances makes the interpretation of pelvic ultrasound more complex than the rather straightforward issue of whether or not an intrauterine pregnancy is present. Nonetheless, when used in conjunction with an appropriate history and physical pelvic examination, ultrasound usually identifies the source of a suspected pelvic problem and often provides a definitive diagnosis.

NORMAL PELVIC ANATOMY

A basic familiarity with the sonographic appearance of the normal pelvis is very useful to the emergency physician, not only for the interpretation of ultrasound images, but also because it leads to a more complete understanding of the female genital and reproductive systems. It is virtually inevitable that the physician's skills, including performance of the routine pelvic examination, will be enhanced by a better understanding of normal pelvic anatomy. This is particularly true if ultrasound is incorporated into the pelvic examination, so that immediate feedback is obtained regarding the location and identity of palpated structures.

As with the suspected ectopic pregnancy, transabdominal pelvic scanning in the non-gravid patient is performed in sagittal and transverse sections with a distended urinary bladder (Figs. 3–39 and 3–40). Once again, the importance of adequate filling of the bladder (usually 300 to 500 mL) cannot be overemphasized, because the bladder provides both an acoustic window for visualization of deeper structures and enhances their visualization by displacing overlying bowel and spreading out the adnexa. The bladder wall is obvious on scanning as a relatively reflective structure that surrounds the extremely sonolucent lumen. The hyperreflective appearance of structures deep to this organ should not be surprising, because they are a direct manifestation of acoustic enhancement (see Chapter 1).

Uterus

The uterine fundus is seen deep to the bladder, the degree of indentation on the bladder surface being variable, depending on the degree of anterior flexion of the uterus, as well as on the degree of filling of the bladder. A slice through the dome-like top of the uterine fundus on transverse scanning would appear more or less oval, although the organ's mobility militates against this appearing perfectly symmetrical in any particular case. The central canal of the uterus appears as a more echogenic structure in the sonolucent endometrium. Considering the pear-shaped structure of the uterus, it is not surprising that the canal is better visualized along its length in the sagittal (longitudinal transvaginal scan) plane (Fig. 3–41). The degree of echogenicity of the endometrium varies with the stage of the menstrual cycle, as does its thickness. It is darkest (more sonolucent) in the early part of the cycle, and becomes thicker and more sonodense (up to 10 mm thick) through

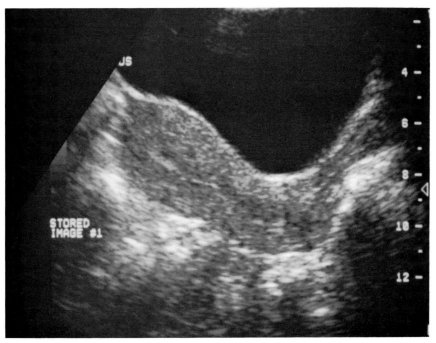

Figure 3–39. Normal sagittal views. Demonstrates the (transabdominal) ultrasound appearance of the normal pelvic anatomy on sagittal section.

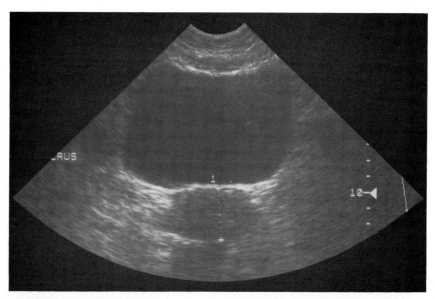

Figure 3–40. Normal transverse view. Demonstrates the (transabdominal) ultrasound appearance of the normal pelvic anatomy on transverse section.

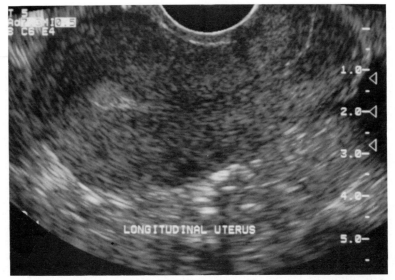

Figure 3–41. Endometrial canal. The echogenic structure in the center of the uterus represents the endometrium on transvaginal scanning. The thickness and brightness of the endometrial echo vary with the menstrual cycle.

ovulation. Indeed, the appearance of the endometrium may be quite variable; during menstruation, it is thin and quite ragged, with some central anechoic areas secondary to the presence of sloughed tissue and blood. It may seem surprising that the normal fallopian tubes are rarely visible during tansabdominal scanning; the proximal tubal lumen may be demonstrated on transvaginal examination, particularly during the menses. Variations in the normal appearance of the uterus may be seen in individuals with a bicornuate uterus; this occurs secondary to a fusion abnormality of the uterus (Fig. 3–42). In addition, nabothian cysts (Fig. 3–43) of the cervix should not be confused with other pathologic conditions.

Muscular Structures

Although not of great importance pathologically, there are four pairs of abdominal muscles that easily can cause confusion with other structures. The ileorectus muscles, with their hyperechoic central region, can easily mimic the

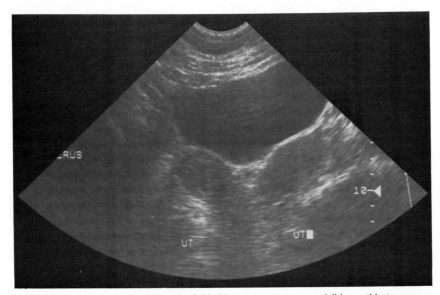

Figure 3–42. Bicornuate uterus. Both "horns" of this bicornuate uterus are visible on this transverse scan.

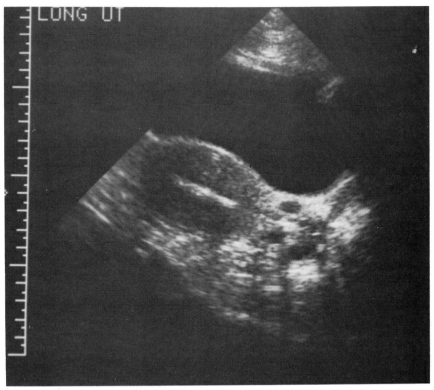

Figure 3–43. Nabothian cysts. These round, anechoic structures within the cervix are not of pathologic significance.

size, shape, and position of the ovaries. The rectus abdominis muscles, piriformis, and the obturator internus are also potential sources of confusion. Various arteries and veins may also be misidentified as other pelvic structures: the internal iliac vein passes just posterior to the ovary (Fig. 3–44) and can appear as a cystic structure in cross section. When viewed in long section, such vessels should be clearly discernible from small cysts and may actually help in locating and identifying structures of interest.

Ovaries

Ovaries are small, $2 \times 2 \times 3$ cm, almond-shaped structures that vary in ultrasound appearance according to the stage of ovulation. In the premenopausal woman, they often appear as rather foamy structures secondary to the presence of multiple follicles. Just prior to ovulation, a single cystic follicle may enlarge as much as 3 cm in diameter before releasing the ovum. This is a unilateral event for each cycle.

Ultrasound scanning can illustrate these follicular cysts in striking detail (Figs. 3–45 and 3–46).

Bowel and Other Structures

The close approximation of the rectosigmoid and the vagina is evident on both rectal and pelvic examinations, and it is not surprising that this portion of bowel should be routinely visualized during ultrasound. The appearance of bowel loops may vary remarkably depending on the particular combination of fluid, formed stool, and gas that they contain. The recognition of bowel is usually not difficult: the gas may produce obvious shadowing, evidence of peristalsis is usually noted, and loops should compress with probe pressure.

It should be clear from the previous discussion that the sonographic appearance of the pelvis is complex and variable. Virtually every organ can vary enormously in size, shape, or location, and frequently in all three. Pelvic ultrasound can help clarify many of the anatomic variations seen in the female patient.

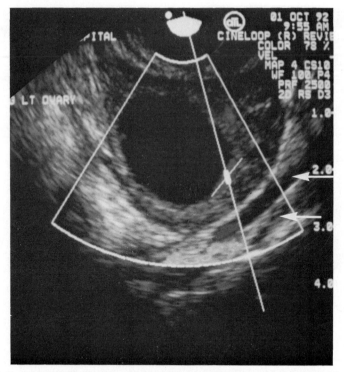

Figure 3-44. Iliac vessels. These vascular structures (*arrows*) are seen just posterior to the ovaries.

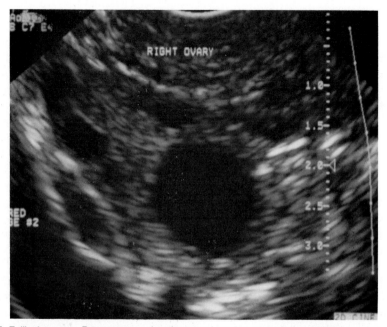

Figure 3-45. Follicular cysts. Demonstrates the ultrasound appearance of normal follicular cysts in the ovary.

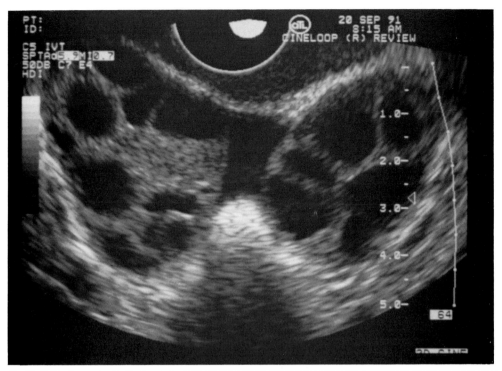

Figure 3–46. Follicular cysts. Patients on progestational agents may be found to have dramatic enlargement in the size of these cystic structures.

SCANNING TECHNIQUES: TRANSABDOMINAL VERSUS TRANSVAGINAL

The implications of transvaginal (endovaginal) scanning are discussed in Chapter 2 because the transvaginal approach has assumed a major role in the diagnosis of suspected ectopic pregnancy. The advantages inherent to the transvaginal approach apply to the nongravid examination as well: specifically, the ability to obtain greater resolution of small structures that are close to the higher resolution probe. The difficulties, however, in a sense are magnified as the smaller field of view and complexities of orientation are applied to the array of pelvic structures, which are far from constant in location, shape, and sonographic appearance. Unlike the traditional sagittal and transverse appearance of the normal pelvis, which soon becomes familiar on viewing transabdominal studies, it is difficult or impossible to obtain a broad overview of the pelvis endovaginally. Rather, the technique is most useful when directed at a small area of interest, such as a region of tenderness or a mass previously found on pelvic examination or transabdominal scan.

Figures 3–47 and 3–48 contrast the ultrasound appearance of a transabdominal and a transvaginal scan of ectopic pregnancies in which the relationship of the adnexal ring in question to the surrounding structures is readily deducible only on transabdominal imaging. At the same time, these figures illustrate the great potential of the transvaginal approach in visualizing tiny structures (Fig. 3–49) that might not be appreciated transabdominally. In addition, the ability to scan patients of any habitus with or without urine in the bladder is often a clear advantage of the transvaginal approach. However, when the source of the symptoms is not well localized, the transvaginal approach is not as satisfactory and may in fact be unsuited to visualization of areas that are out in the adnexa or in the lower abdomen. For many general emergency department studies, the transabdominal examination may be preferred and may even be required. When the area of interest is localized and, particularly, when transabdominal scanning does not provide detailed

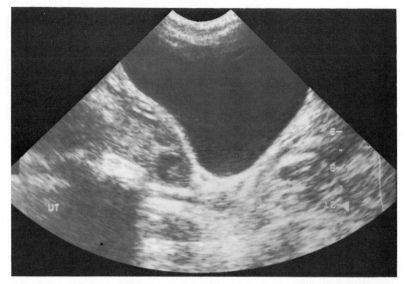

Figure 3–47. Ectopic pregnancy. Demonstrates the transabdominal view of an ectopic pregnancy where the surrounding structures may be easily identified. (From Jehle D, Braen R, Krause R: Ectopic pregnancy. Emerg Med Clin North Am 12:55–71, 1994.)

enough information to resolve a clinical question, it makes sense to perform a transvaginal scan of that region.

PELVIC MASSES

It is not uncommon that a pelvic mass or, more ambiguously, "an abnormal fullness" is found on pelvic or abdominal examination; at times, these masses may be noted on plain radiographs or CT as well.

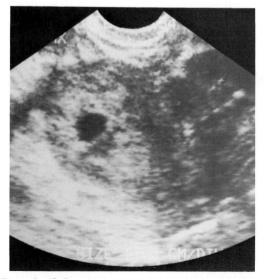

Figure 3–48. Ectopic pregnancy. Illustrates the adnexal ring of an ectopic pregnancy with better resolution, but without the field of view of Figure 3–47.

Simple Cysts

It must be remembered that in premenopausal women, a single ovarian follicle may enlarge 100 times in volume, up to about 3 cm, over a 10-day period in the mid- and late follicular phases of the cycle. These follicular cysts (Figs. 3–45 and 3–46) normally resolve after ovulation. At times, however, the resulting corpus luteum can persist and enlarge to 10 cm in size. These functional cysts may be symptomatic and easily palpated on pelvic examination; however, they ordinarily regress over a period of 2 months without intervention. The ultrasound appearance of a corpus luteum cyst is quite varied and reflects hemorrhage, clot formation, retraction, and resorption (Fig. 3–50). Such findings require no immediate intervention, but follow-up ultrasound is indicated to document regression of the structure. For those cysts that persist more than 8 weeks, needle aspiration or surgical removal should be considered. Other simple cysts may form in the round ligament or other adnexal structures (Figs. 3–51 and 3–52); they may be symptomatic or found incidentally on pelvic examination. Again, no intervention other than follow-up is required.

Complex Cysts

Other masses are found, on ultrasound examination, to have septations or other internal structures. These are of greater concern in that

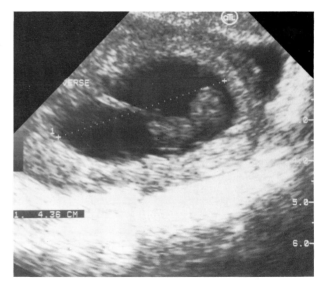

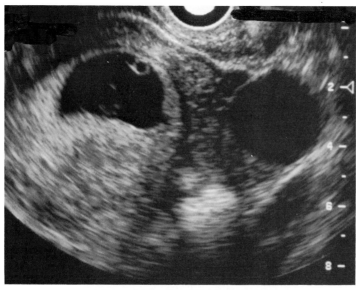

Figure 3–49. Ectopic pregnancy. This illustrates the detail that may be visualized on transvaginal scanning. Note the absence of surrounding myometrium and the small amount of (dark) free pelvic fluid. (From Jehle D, Braen R, Krause R: Ectopic pregnancy. Emerg Med Clin North Am 12:55–71, 1994.)

Figure 3–50. Corpus luteum cyst. This demonstrates an intrauterine pregnancy with a visible yolk sac (*left*) and a large adjacent anechoic structure that represents a corpus luteum cyst (*right*). The corpus luteum cyst usually disappears before the end of the second trimester of pregnancy.

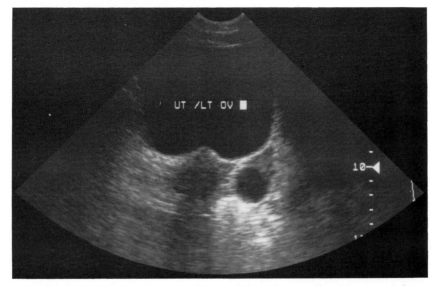

Figure 3–51. Cystic adnexal mass. Note the appearance of an anechoic ovarian cyst. Note the presence of posterior enhancement.

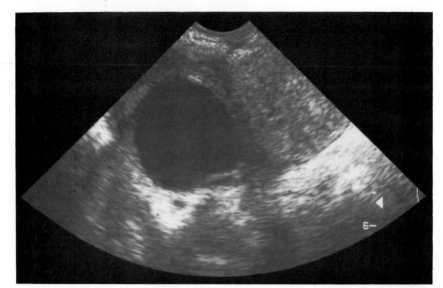

Figure 3-52. Cystic adnexal mass. Note the appearance of an anechoic ovarian cyst with posterior enhancement.

they have an increased chance of representing a malignancy or a tubo-ovarian abscess. In general, combined cystic and solid masses require a tissue diagnosis in order to exclude malignancy. Figures 3-53 and 3-54 illustrate the sonographic appearance of complex masses.

Solid Masses

There are a host of malignancies that may present in the pelvis as a solid mass. Potentially, all require tissue diagnosis.

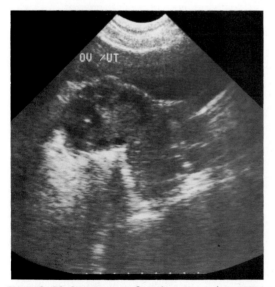

Figure 3-53. Complex cyst. Complex masses demonstrate both cystic and echogenic components.

Endometriosis

For reasons that are unclear, ectopic endometrium can implant throughout the pelvis and even extend through abdomen and thorax. This tissue remains hormonally responsive and undergoes bleeding and proliferation in accord with the woman's menstrual cycle. In the emergency department, affected patients complain of pain that is cyclical in nature, and evidence of scarring or infertility may be present as well. Endometriomas are hollow collections of such tissue that are filled with blood and have long been dubbed "chocolate cysts." These most often form in the ovary but can occur most anywhere and can rarely create a true emergency by rupturing or causing the ovary to undergo torsion.

Fibroids

Leiomyomas represent the most common tumors of women (Fig. 3-55). These benign nodules can undergo several forms of degeneration, leading to different ultrasound appearances. When degeneration occurs, the center of the leiomyoma appears more lucent than the exterior and, with an improper gain setting, can be mistaken for a cystic structure. Other leiomyomas do in fact undergo liquefaction necrosis. Fibroids all arise in the uterine wall, but they assume a wide variety of shapes and locations. Ultrasound examination can strongly suggest the diagnosis.

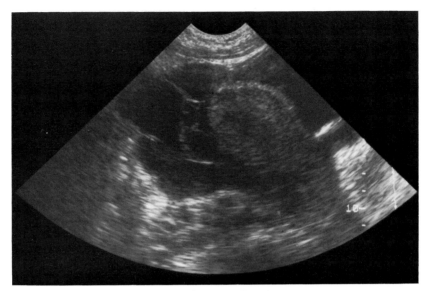

Figure 3-54. Complex adnexal mass.

Pelvic Inflammatory Disease

Pelvic inflammatory disease (PID) is a ubiquitous emergency department ailment that can sometimes be suggested but not diagnosed by ultrasound. Evidence of fallopian tube dysfunction and obstruction cannot be visualized, but when this disease progresses untreated, a tubo-ovarian abscess (TOA) may develop (Fig. 3-56). The documentation of a TOA mandates hospitalization, intravenous therapy, and sometimes surgery as well. Pelvic ultrasound plays a key role in making the diagnosis of a TOA.

Lost Intrauterine Device

Although intrauterine devices (IUDs) have become much less common as a form of contraception in recent years, they are still used by a significant number of women. A fairly common event is that a usually evident string can no longer be felt or seen; the problem of a lost IUD exists. Appearances of the different IUDs are well recognized on ultrasound. Figure 3-57 illustrates a sagittal view of a popular IUD located centrally in the uterus. Transabdominal and transvaginal ultrasound can detect IUDs with a high degree of accuracy and, in the case of concomitant pregnancy, significant risks exist both with attempted extraction and conservative therapy. The physician must remember that the presence of an IUD makes the possibility of ectopic pregnancy more likely.

SECOND AND THIRD TRIMESTER PREGNANCY

The primary role of emergency department ultrasound in the second and third trimesters of pregnancy is to document fetal viability (Fig. 3-58). However, some basic familiarity with the ultrasound appearance of the normal fetus later in pregnancy enhances the emergency physician's ability to perform satisfactory scanning of these patients (Figs. 3-59 to 3-65). Following the first trimester of pregnancy, measurement of the biparietal diameter replaces crown-rump length as the method of choice for estimating gestational age (Fig. 3-66). Femur length, head circumference, and abdominal circumference are alternative methods that are regularly used to calculate fetal age.

Ultrasound is frequently used to detect fetal anomalies (Figs. 3-67 and 3-68). Sonography is also helpful in evaluating the patient with third trimester vaginal bleeding for placenta previa (Fig. 3-69) or abruptio placentae (Fig. 3-70). It should be noted that the ultrasound evaluation does not replace cardiotocographic monitoring (maternal-fetal monitoring of at least 4 hours) of the third trimester pregnancy with significant abdominal trauma.

Text continued on page 184

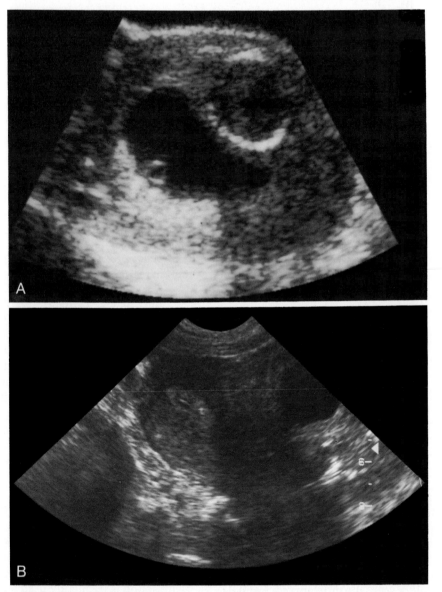

Figure 3–55. *A* and *B*, Fibroids. *A*, The appearance of a leiomyoma (fibroid) adjacent to an intrauterine pregnancy. This fibroid has an echogenic border; however, fibroids have a wide variety of ultrasound appearances. *B*, An echogenic fibroid in the posterior portion of the uterus of a nonpregnant patient.

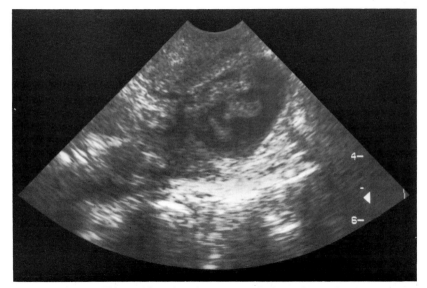

Figure 3–56. Tubo-ovarian abscess. This complex adnexal mass proved to be a tubo-ovarian abscess in a patient with pelvic inflammatory disease.

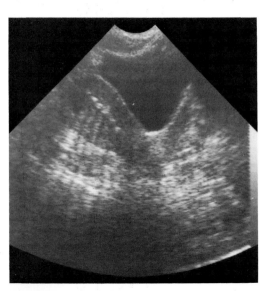

Figure 3–57. Intrauterine device (IUD). This sagittal view demonstrates ultrasound appearance of an IUD located centrally in the uterus.

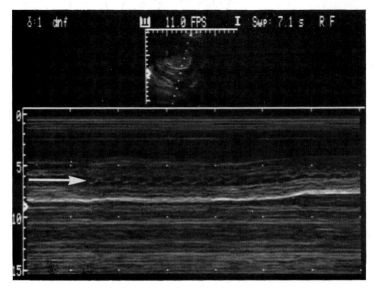

Figure 3–58. Fetal viability. This M-mode image documents the presence and the rate of fetal cardiac activity (*arrow*) plotted against time.

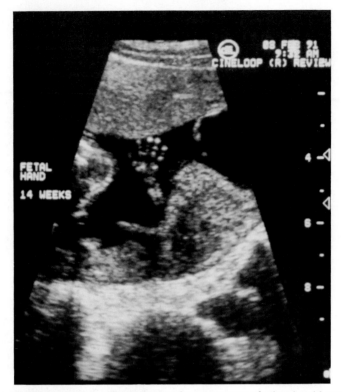

Figure 3–59. Normal fetus. Demonstrates the appearance of a hand at 14 weeks.

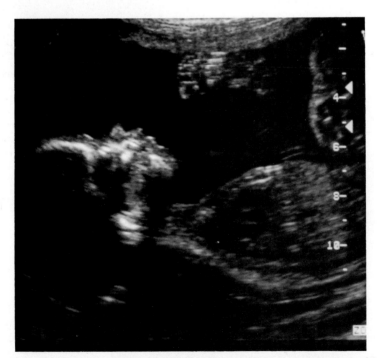

Figure 3–60. Normal fetus. Demonstrates a profile of the fetal face. Note the foot anterior to the body of the fetus in this image.

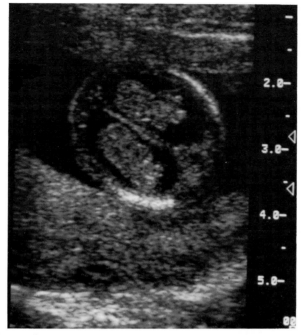

Figure 3-61. Normal fetus. Illustrates the appearance of the choroid plexus in a 12.5 week fetus.

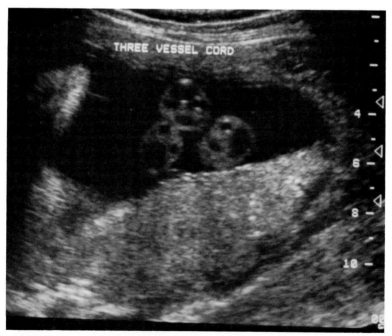

Figure 3-62. Normal fetus. Demonstrates the appearance of the umbilical cord when imaged in cross section (×3). The two umbilical arteries and single umbilical vein are easily visualized within the cord.

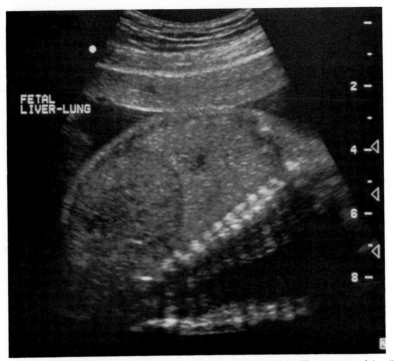

Figure 3–63. Normal fetus. Demonstrates the appearance of the fetal lung and liver. The contour of the diaphragm makes it clear that the lung is in the right portion of the image.

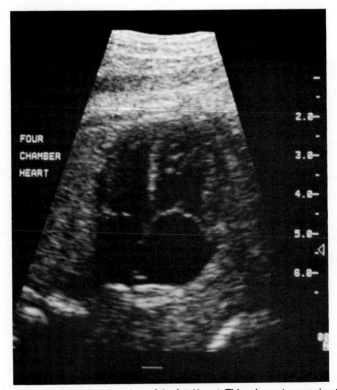

Figure 3–64. Normal fetus. A normal, four-chamber view of the fetal heart. This rules out approximately 95% of fetal cardiac anomalies.

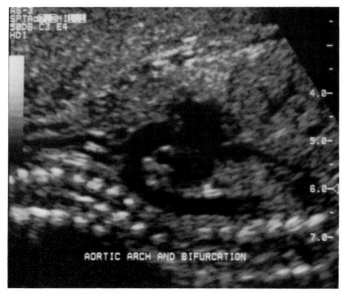

Figure 3–65. Normal fetus. Illustrates the aortic arch and some of its branches anterior to the fetal spine. The ossification centers of the spine do not fuse in utero, leading to a "railroad track" appearance.

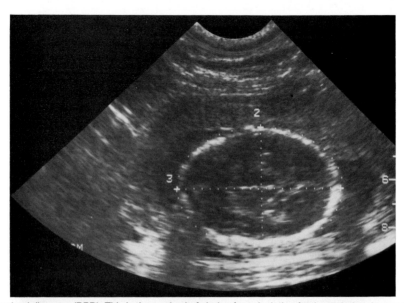

Figure 3–66. Biparietal diameter (BPD). This is the method of choice for calculating fetal age during the second and third trimester of pregnancy. BPD should be measured at the level of the thalamus (paired central anechoic structures). Head circumference is also being measured in this image.

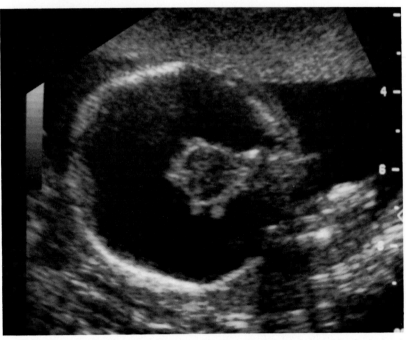

Figure 3–67. Holoprosencephaly. This refers to a disorder resulting from the failure of normal forebrain development. There is minimal remaining cerebral tissue, which is surrounded by a large monoventricular cavity.

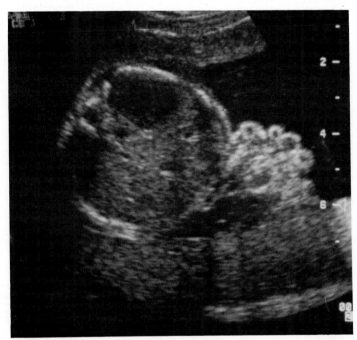

Figure 3–68. Gastroschisis. This is a defect involving all layers of the abdominal wall. There is evisceration of multiple loops of bowel outside of the true abdominal cavity.

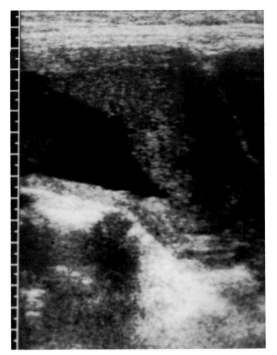

Figure 3–69. Placenta previa. The placenta covers the entire cervical os. Clinically, this presents with painless vaginal bleeding in the third trimester of pregnancy.

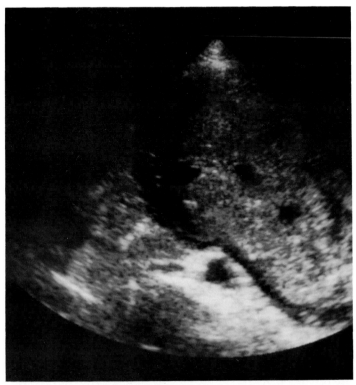

Figure 3–70. Abruptio placentae. The anechoic space with scattered focal echogenicities represents blood (and clot) from premature separation of the placenta from the uterus. Most women with abruptions present with painful vaginal bleeding.

Other Cardiac Applications

David Plummer, MD

USES OF TWO-DIMENSIONAL ECHOCARDIOGRAPHY

Besides the two primary cardiac indications (cardiac tamponade and electromechanical dissociation [EMD]) discussed in Chapter 2 there are several other emergency department uses of two-dimensional (2-D) echocardiography that merit consideration. Although not considered primary, in some emergency departments they have already become routine. At this time there are at least two good reasons to expect that the use of these bedside applications will increase rapidly. First is the very nature of acute and serious cardiac disease of almost any type. Whether the underlying process is ischemic or traumatic, the criterion of a time-critical nature is usually fulfilled. Second, the ability to affect the course of acute cardiac disease by early intervention (thrombolysis, angioplasty, surgery, and mechanical support) has been arguably the single most dramatic medical advance of the past decade. Each of these interventions may cause serious complications, often death, if instituted inappropriately; all require rapid anatomic or physiologic data that cannot be obtained with traditional laboratory and x-ray studies. Early diagnosis and intervention in ischemic heart disease have moved rapidly from the intensive care unit to the cardiac catheterization laboratory and now to the emergency department. Accordingly, our cardiology colleagues have often been the most positive and potent advocates for the adoption of 2-D echocardiography as an emergency department tool.

Sonographic Considerations

Performance and interpretation of even limited echocardiographic examination require a body of functional knowledge and experience that takes time to acquire. For each condition discussed below, identification and assessment of cardiac chambers and related structure are necessary, as is a judgment regarding wall motion. Both goals require that certain standard views or windows be used during cardiac scanning. These are summarized in Table 3–1 and discussed in detail below. It should be noted that:

1. The usual references to transverse, sagittal, and coronal are not used
2. The usual conventions regarding orientation of the marker groove do not apply
3. The marker groove continues to point to the left side of the screen
4. The physician must know a selection of standard windows.

Each window views the heart from a different perspective, and each has both advantages and disadvantages. The following is a selection of the standard windows used for a limited examination.

The *subcostal window* often provides the most significant information for a single-view examination. To obtain this view, place the transducer at the left infracostal margin at the level of the xiphoid with the beam aimed at the left shoulder (Fig. 3–71). The examiner can slightly tilt or rotate the transducer in order to obtain the desired view. The structures closest to the transducer appear nearest the top of the display. With the patient supine, the most anterior structure is a small amount of hepatic parenchyma, followed by the right-sided cardiac chambers (Figs. 3–72 and 3–73). The anterior and posterior aspects of the pericardium appear as single, bright reflecting surfaces. Separation of these bright echoes represents a separation of

Table 3–1. STANDARD CARDIAC WINDOWS*

Standard View	Probe Position/Direction	Advantages
Subcostal (SC)	Left intercostal margin at xiphoid Beam toward left shoulder	Readily accessible; screen for fluid, wall motion, and chamber size; supine position adequate
Left parasternal long axis (LPLA)	Left parasternal 2–4 inches Beam toward back	Easily interpreted; proximal aorta, left ventricle, left atrium well seen
Left parasternal short axis (LPSA)	Left parasternal 2–4 inches Beam varies with level (right shoulder to left hip)	Mitral and aortic valves well seen; global LV function visualized
Apical	Cardiac apex Beam toward right shoulder	Easily interpreted; all 4 chambers seen; contractility, size, and fluid visualized

*If the standard abdominal ultrasound machine "set up" is maintained, the marker dot points toward 4 o'clock for LPLA, 8 o'clock for LPSA and apical, and 8 to 9 o'clock for SC.

the visceral and parietal pericardium, usually by fluid (Fig. 3–74). Although a small amount of fluid is normal in the pericardial sac, any separation anteriorly (the nondependent portion with the patient supine) represents an abnormal collection, frequently a pericardial effusion or hemopericardium. One can quickly view the abdominal aorta from the same transducer position by simply tilting and rotating the transducer. The subcostal view has several advantages as a starting point. It quickly screens for mechanical activity, pericardial fluid, and gross assessment of global and regional wall motion abnormalities and provides a four-chamber view in order to assess the relative size of the ventricles. The physician can readily obtain this view in supine, noncompliant, and critically ill patients. A limited, goal-directed examination may be obtained from the subcostal window within 1 minute.

The *left parasternal views* result from placing the transducer in the left parasternal area between the second and the fourth intercostal spaces (Fig. 3–75). Rotating the transducer gives either a left parasternal short-axis (LPSA) or left parasternal long-axis view (LPLA). For the LPLA, the plane of the beam is parallel to a line drawn from the right shoulder to the left hip (Figs. 3–76 and 3–77). This view allows visualization of the aortic valve, proximal ascending aorta, and a good assessment of left ventricular size. Rotating the transducer so that the plane of the beam is perpendicular to the long axis of the heart (i.e., toward the left

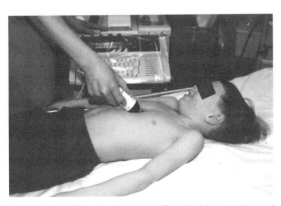

Figure 3–71. Transducer position for obtaining a subcostal echocardiogram.

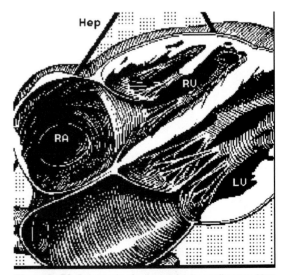

Figure 3–72. Schematic of subcostal echocardiogram. Hep, hepatic parenchyma; LV, left ventricle; RA, right atrium; RV, right ventricle.

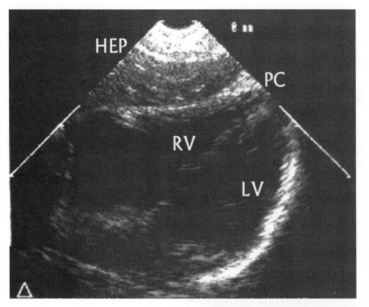

Figure 3–73. Normal subcostal echocardiogram. Hep, hepatic parenchyma; LV, left ventricle; PC, pericardium; RV, right ventricle.

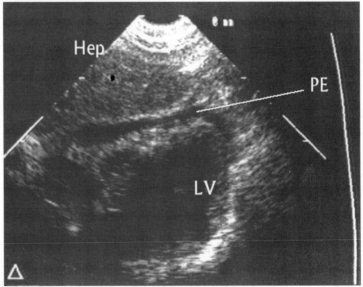

Figure 3–74. Subcostal echocardiogram demonstrating pericardial effusion. Hep, hepatic parenchyma; LV, left ventricle; PE, pericardial effusion.

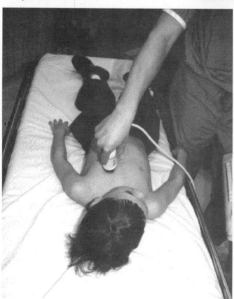

Figure 3–75. Transducer position for obtaining a left parasternal window. This position is used for both the long- and short-axis variations.

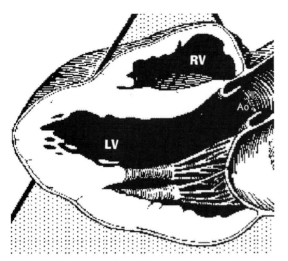

Figure 3-76. Schematic of left parasternal long-axis window. Ao, aortic outflow; LV, left ventricle; RV, right ventricle.

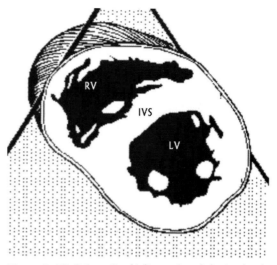

Figure 3-78. Schematic of left parasternal short-axis window. IVS, intraventricular septum; LV, left ventricle; RV, right ventricle.

shoulder) reveals the LPSA (Figs. 3–78 and 3–79). By tilting the transducer, one can visualize from the apex through the mitral valve to the aortic valve. Both of the left parasternal windows may require positioning the patient in the left lateral decubitus position, which eliminates interposed lung between the transducer and the heart. These views may be difficult to obtain in a noncompliant, critically ill patient.

The *apical view* results from placing the transducer directly over the point of maximum impulse (the apex) with the beam directed to the right shoulder (Fig. 3–80). The operator must tilt and rotate the transducer to get the desired view (Figs. 3–81 and 3–82). The apical view allows for assessment of chamber size and location of intracavitary masses. It also frequently

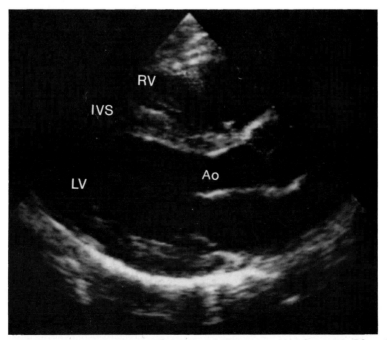

Figure 3-77. Normal left parasternal long-axis view. IVS, intraventricular septum; LV, left ventricle; PC, pericardium; RV, right ventricle.

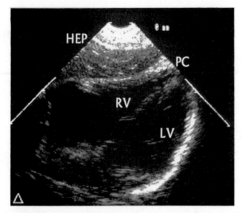

Figure 3-79. Left parasternal short-axis window. LV, left ventricle; PC, pericardium; RV, right ventricle.

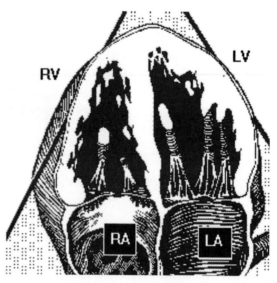

Figure 3-81. Schematic of the apical window. LA, left atrium; LV, left ventricle; RA, right atrium; RV, right ventricle.

requires positioning in the left lateral decubitus position.

These four windows and views represent only a sampling of those used in a formal echocardiographic examination. Although it is necessary to know these standard windows, an echocardiographic examination is interactive and the operator must be prepared to adapt the transducer position during the examination. Often, the emergency physician need not perform each of these windows in order to answer the limited clinical question. The best window for any examination is the one that gives the desired information.

Clinical Considerations

Besides the indications outlined in Chapter 2, the clinical situations in which emergency department 2-D echocardiography is likely to be useful are listed in Table 3–2; each is considered separately. Even more so than most such classifications, there is great overlap among the categories, because the two common symptoms (pain and shock) that prompt investigation are common to most types of acute heart disease. In addition, there are many other clinical situations that may prompt echocardiographic evaluation, including questions raised by unexpected findings on physical examination, electrocardiogram (ECG), or radiography (rubs, clicks, peripheral emboli, paradoxical emboli, endocarditis, transplant rejection, electrical alternans, low voltage, enlarged cardiac silhouette, and others). In some of these cases, the clinical condition will be such that bedside ultrasound examination rather than (or before) referral for formal echocardiographic examination is appropriate.

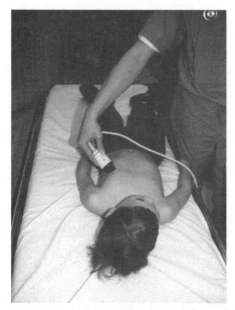

Figure 3-80. Transducer position for obtaining an apical window.

Table 3-2. CLINICAL SITUATIONS IN WHICH TWO-DIMENSIONAL ECHOCARDIOGRAPHY IS USEFUL

Hypotension of unknown cause
Cardiac trauma—either blunt or penetrating
Ischemic heart disease
Disease of the great vessels
Iatrogenic: complications of procedures

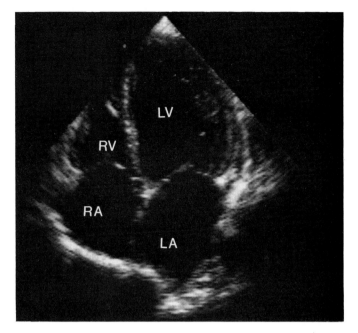

Figure 3-82. Echocardiogram from the apical window. LA, left atrium; LV, left ventricle; RA, right atrium; RV, right ventricle.

HYPOTENSION OF UNKNOWN CAUSE

Patients frequently arrive at the emergency department with hypotension and shock. Successful resuscitation depends on rapid treatment directed at the primary hemodynamic alteration. The physical examination is often both nonspecific and insensitive in detecting the underlying hemodynamic state. Invasive diagnostic testing (intraarterial catheterization, central venous pressure measurements, and pulmonary artery catheterization) is costly, time consuming, and not easily performed in many emergency departments. In this setting, bedside 2-D echocardiography performed via a single window may rapidly and specifically guide initial resuscitation efforts. By assessing the global motion of the heart and the chamber size, the patient can often be quickly assigned to one of four hemodynamic categories: (1) cardiogenic shock (left ventricular dysfunction), (2) hypovolemia, (3) right ventricular dysfunction, and (4) cardiac tamponade.

Patients with *cardiogenic shock* (from cardiomyopathy, ischemic heart disease, etc.) display marked global wall motion abnormalities on 2-D echocardiography. Patients with acute myocardial infarction as the cause for hypotension usually display discrete left ventricular dysfunction. Echocardiography aids in defining

both the cause and possible therapy of the patient's shock. Serial examinations allow immediate feedback about the impact of fluid and drug administrations. The extreme case is represented by the patient erroneously thought to be in EMD (see Chapter 2) in whom wall and valve motion are clearly present, but perfusion pressure is severely compromised. These patients require aggressive inotropic and mechanical support.

Patients who are *hypovolemic* usually display a hyperkinetic heart with small right-sided chambers. This results from either absolute hypovolemia, as in hemorrhagic shock, or from relative hypovolemia, as in states of reduced afterload (i.e., early shock with preserved cardiac function). In such cases, the initial therapeutic measures must include vigorous fluid resuscitation, and serial 2-D echocardiography examination can help guide therapy. Unexplained hypovolemia of this degree may be due to simple dehydration, but unsuspected trauma and occult exsanguination from aneurysms and grafts must always be considered.

Patients with *pulmonary embolism* who present hypotensive often have 2-D echocardiography consistent with acute right ventricular outflow obstruction. These patients display a vigorously beating left ventricle with a large, hypodynamic, thin-walled right ventricle (Figs. 3-83 and 3-84). Additionally, they may dis-

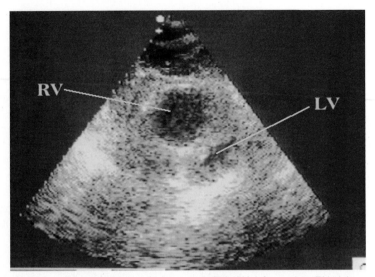

Figure 3–83. Subcostal echocardiogram in acute pulmonary embolism. LV, left ventricle; RV, right ventricle. Note massive dilation of RV.

play paradoxical interventricular septal motion, indicating high right ventricular pressures, and concurrent right atrial thrombus. The 2-D echocardiography profile in massive right ventricular infarct is similar. In both cases, early bedside diagnosis may allow for the rapid institution of thrombolytic therapy and volume replacement.

The final 2-D echocardiography pattern seen with hypotension is that of *cardiac tamponade*, discussed in Chapter 2. In cases where hypotension is found to be associated with both a pericardial effusion and diastolic collapse of the right-sided chambers, the diagnosis is firmly established. The underlying cause, which may be

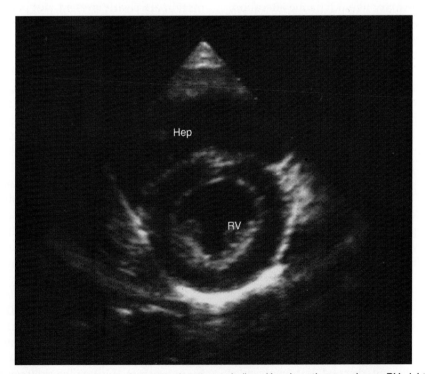

Figure 3–84. Subcostal echocardiogram in acute pulmonary embolism. Hep, hepatic parenchyma; RV, right ventricle. Note massive dilation of RV.

anything from cardiac rupture to viral pericarditis, may not be evident. In cases where the only definite finding is the pericardial effusion and the diagnosis of tamponade is not established, it must be remembered that many causes of pericardial fluid (myopericarditis, severe congestive heart failure [CHF], uremia, etc.) may also be associated with hypotension without tamponade.

CARDIAC TRAUMA

Penetrating Injury

Historically, most patients with major cardiac injuries die at the scene. Many factors, including improved emergency medicine systems and the increasing incidence of urban violence, have greatly increased the number of salvageable patients who present to emergency departments with penetrating injury and cardiac trauma. It is firmly established that rapid diagnosis and treatment of penetrating cardiac injury is an independent determinant of survival of these patients.

Unfortunately, the signs and symptoms on physical examination are both nonspecific and insensitive and often are recognized only when catastrophic deterioration occurs. Traditional imaging techniques (CT and angiography) employed for diagnosis of penetrating cardiac injury are often not immediately available to such patients. However, a limited 2-D echocardiography bedside examination can quite readily be performed in approximately 1 minute, independent of patient compliance.

Hemopericardium is the most common visible feature of penetrating cardiac injury and presents as an echo-free space within the pericardium (Fig. 3–85). This anechoic appearance occurs early on if there is brisk bleeding or later due to liquefication of the pericardial hematoma from defibrination of blood. The latter regularly occurs in subacute and chronic hemopericardium. In acute hemopericardium, however, there may be insufficient time for defibrination to occur; as a result, the hemopericardium can organize and partially clot, resulting in a pericardial hematoma. Such hematomas appear diffusely echogenic instead of echo-free (Figs. 3–86, 3–87, and 3–88), and the hematoma may even be isodense to the myocardium, making ultrasound diagnosis difficult. Any intrapericardial collections, whether echo-free or echo-dense, in the setting of penetrating injury to the thorax or upper abdomen are considered to represent penetrating cardiac injury. Rarely, a patient with cardiac penetration has a normal-appearing echocardiogram if the hemopericardium decompresses into the thorax. Also uncommonly, patients may display pneumopericardium, pericardial foreign bodies, or pseudoaneurysm formation.

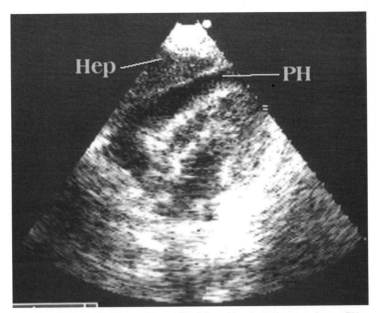

Figure 3–85. Subcostal echocardiogram in penetrating cardiac injury. Hep, hepatic parenchyma; PH, pericardial hematoma.

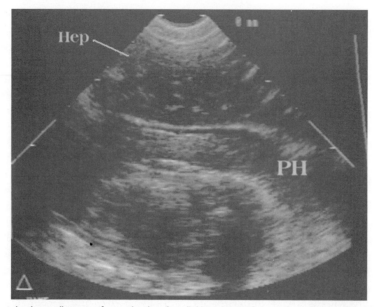

Figure 3–86. Subcostal echocardiogram of organized pericardial hematoma from penetrating cardiac injury. Note the echogenic characteristics of organized pericardial blood. Hep, hepatic parenchyma; PH, pericardial hematoma.

Blunt Injury

Patients sustaining blunt chest injury may suffer cardiac contusion, myocardial hematoma, or cardiac rupture. Cardiac contusion, although variably defined, may lead to arrhythmias, pump failure, or thromboembolism. Concurrent multisystem injury often obscures the early diagnosis. Laboratory diagnosis, including standard and right precordial ECG, creatine phosphokinase-MB (CPK-MB) fractionation,

first-pass radionuclide angiography, technetium-99m pyrophosphate, thallium-201, and single photon emission computed tomography (SPECT) scanning, is technically difficult and has insufficient sensitivity or specificity to serve as a standard. However, 2-D echocardiography, which can be performed at the bedside, is quite sensitive and specific; up to 25% of blunt trauma victims not suspected clinically of cardiac contusion have 2-D echocardiographic evidence of wall motion abnormalities consistent

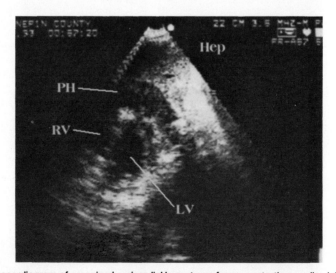

Figure 3–87. Subcostal echocardiogram of organized pericardial hematoma from penetrating cardiac injury. Note the echogenic characteristics of organized pericardial blood. PH, pericardial hematoma; RV, right ventricle; LV, left ventricle; Hep, hepatic parenchyma.

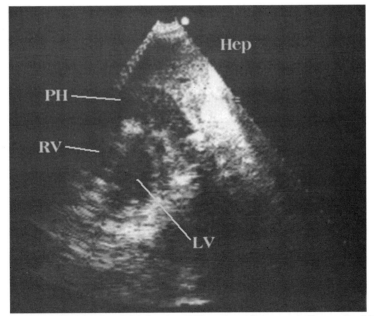

Figure 3-88. Subcostal echocardiogram of organized pericardial hematoma from penetrating cardiac injury. This echo was obtained within minutes of injury and shows echogenic characteristics of organized pericardial blood. Hep, hepatic parenchyma; LV, left ventricle; PH, pericardial hematoma; RV, right ventricle.

with this diagnosis, and a pericardial effusion is often also present.

The whole issue is clouded by the lack of a gold standard and by the growing consensus that *clinically significant* cardiac contusion is usually evident (e.g., arrhythmias, hypotension, CHF) early in the resuscitation. Deceleration injuries most commonly contuse the right ventricle because it is the most anterior aspect of the heart. Therefore, 2-D echocardiographic evidence of right ventricular dilation and dysfunction strongly supports the diagnosis of contusion. Although there is debate regarding the significance of isolated cardiac contusion on outcome, it is an important diagnosis to make in the hemodynamically unstable patient. Clearly, 2-D echocardiography in this setting can aid in directing resuscitating methods, including inotropic agents and intraaortic balloon pump therapy. Perhaps just as importantly, it can help avoid these measures in the hypovolemic patient.

Rarely, patients with blunt chest trauma arrive with cardiac rupture. This injury probably has the same time–mortality profile as traumatic aortic rupture, with most patients dying at the scene. However, in the patients entering the emergency medicine system alive, survival re-

quires rapid diagnosis and treatment. Usually, the pericardial sac contains the rupture, and these patients have hemopericardium and some degree of cardiac tamponade. This diagnosis should always be suspected when hemopericardium presents in the setting of blunt trauma. Rarely, an extrapericardial mediastinal hematoma with cardiac compression has a similar appearance to a ruptured heart.

ISCHEMIC HEART DISEASE

Evaluation of patients with possible ischemic heart disease is a common task for the emergency physician. Although admission rates are high for these patients, missed acute myocardial infarction (AMI) continues to result in significant mortality and liability. Interventional therapies such as thrombolysis, angioplasty, and surgery are now important options in the management of patients with AMI who require rapid and specific diagnosis. Two-dimensional echocardiography performed at the bedside offers an additional noninvasive tool for evaluation of chest pain patients. Ischemic myocardium is uniformly hypokinetic or dyskinetic, resulting in wall motion abnormalities on 2-D echocardiography that aid in the immediate diagnosis of ischemic heart disease. Although formal echocardiography uses a complicated scoring system to describe motion over rigidly defined anatomic segments of the heart, 2-D echocardiography can be used as a screening tool to assess qualitatively global and regional wall motion. When used similarly in the intensive care setting, adequate examinations for wall motion abnormalities were accomplished in over 92% of patients with hand-held 2-D echocardiography. The technique may be particularly helpful in patients with a nondiagnostic ECG who have no known cardiac disease. Although a normal study in such a patient is of limited value, an abnormal study establishes the diagnosis of cardiac disease of indeterminate age, which often mandates admission and cardiac work-up.

Physicians may use bedside 2-D echocardiography in patients who are candidates for thrombolysis in order to exclude other causes for chest pain. This is particularly important in patients who present with mechanical catastrophes such as myocardial pseudoaneurysm, myocardial rupture, and aortic dissection. Although such cases are uncommon, they represent immediate surgical indications and thrombolytic contraindications. Each of these conditions presents as an echogenic pericardial mass, usually a hemopericardium, often with acute or subacute cardiac tamponade. In addition, patients with pericarditis may present with pain and ECGs that mimic AMI. Thrombolytic therapy in this setting has special risks. All patients with the unexpected finding of pericardial fluid by 2-D echocardiography should have thrombolysis withheld until the cause is clearly established.

DISEASE OF THE GREAT VESSELS

Aortography and contrast CT are the two traditional tools used to diagnose acute thoracic dissections. Clearly, 2-D echocardiography and, specifically, transesophageal 2-D echocardiography (TEE) are both sensitive and specific for this diagnosis, perhaps more so than any other technique. In some centers, TEE is now commonly performed by cardiologists at the bedside in patients with suspected aortic dissection. Retrograde dissection with rupture into the pericardial space is the major cause of early mortality in dissection. Therefore, the patients at greatest immediate risk present with hemopericardium, easily seen on standard transthoracic examination. Additionally, the left parasternal views provide an indication of aortic diameter, which generally dilates in type I and type II dissections. Patients with either hemopericardium or enlarged aortic outflow require immediate cardiothoracic consultation.

IATROGENIC (PROCEDURAL) COMPLICATIONS

When a patient decompensates during or following an invasive vascular procedure, the physician can use echocardiography to rapidly screen for inadvertent cardiac penetration with tamponade after central venous pressure (CVP), Swan, or intravenous pacer placement. The same is true following intracardiac injection or attempted pericardiocentesis. Pneumothorax and hemothorax are other complications that may be suspected or confirmed based on ultrasound findings. Patients who experience hemodynamic decompensation after thrombolytic therapy may have evidence of pericardial tamponade or intrathoracic hemorrhage.

SUMMARY

The use of cardiac ultrasound for the types of clinical problems discussed here has much to offer the emergency department physician that is not often available through other means. This is particularly true in highly morbid conditions such as penetrating trauma, AMI, and severe shock of uncertain cause. Rapid changes in these areas make it possible that one or more such indications may be accepted as primary applications in the future. All these uses, however, require a degree of knowledge and experience that is significantly greater than that required for the current primary indications of cardiac tamponade and EMD.

SELECTED READINGS

Cardiac Applications

Buda A: The role of echocardiography in the evaluation of mechanical complications of acute myocardial infarction. Circulation 1991;84(suppl I):109–121.

Come PC: Echocardiographic recognition of pulmonary arterial disease and determination of its course. Am J Med 1988;84:384–394.

Conrad SA, Byrnes TJ: Diastolic collapse of the left and right ventricles in cardiac tamponade. Am Heart J 1988;115: 475–478.

Goldberger JJ, Hemelman RB, Wolfe CL, et al: Right ventricular infarction: Recognition and assessment of its hemodynamic significance by two-dimensional echocardiography. J Am Soc Echocardiogr 1991;4:140–146.

Henry WL, Demaria A, Gramiak R, et al: Report of the American Society of Echocardiography, Committee on Nomenclature and Standards in Two-Dimensional Echocardiography. Circulation 1980;62:212–217.

Oh JK, Miller FA, Shub C, et al: Evaluation of acute chest pain syndromes by two-dimensional echocardiography: its potential application in the selection of patients for acute reperfusion therapy. Mayo Clin Proc 1987;62:59–66.

Oh JK, Shub C, Miller FA, et al: Role of two-dimensional echocardiography in the emergency room. Echocardiography 1985;2:217–226.

Pandian NG, Kusay BS: Use of emergency echocardiography. Cardiology 1989;11:119.

Peels CH, Visser CA, Funke Kupper AJ, et al: Usefulness of two-dimensional echocardiography for immediate detection of myocardial ischemia in the emergency room. Am J Cardiol 1990;65:687–691.

Pierard LA, Albert A, Henrard L, et al: Incidence and significance of pericardial effusion in acute myocardial infarction as determined by two-dimensional echocardiography. J Am Coll Cardiol 1986;8:517–520.

Porembka DT, Hoit BD: Transesophageal echocardiography in the intensive care patient. Crit Care Med 1991; 19:826–835.

Prop RL, Winters WL: Clinical competence in adult echocardiography. Circulation 1990;81:2032–2036.

Sabia P, Afrookteh A, Touchstone DA, et al: Value of regional wall motion abnormality in the emergency room diagnosis of acute myocardial infarction: A prospective study using two-dimensional echocardiography. Circulation 1991;84:85–92.

Schiavone WA, Chumrawi BK, Catalano DR, et al: The use of echocardiography in the emergency management of nonpenetrating traumatic cardiac rupture. Ann Emerg Med 191;20:1248–1250.

Seward JB, Khandheria BK, Oh JK, et al: Transesophageal echocardiography: Technique, anatomic correlations, implementation and clinical applications. Mayo Clin Proc 1988;63:649–680.

Shenoy MM, Dhala A, Khanna A: Transesophageal echocardiography in emergency medicine and critical care. Am J Emerg Med 1991;9:580–587.

Wilson DB, Vacek JL: Echocardiography: Basics for the primary care physician. Postgrad Med 1990;87:191–202.

Texts

Modern echocardiographic texts deal largely with techniques and conditions that are not likely to be explored in the emergency department. For greater exposure to descriptions and images relative to cardiac tamponade and electromechanical dissociation, any general text that includes basic echocardiographic windows is certainly adequate.

Feigenbaum H: Echocardiography, 4th ed. Philadelphia: Lea & Febiger, 1986.

Fleischer AC, James AE: Diagnostic Sonography: Principles and Clinical Applications. Philadelphia: W. B. Saunders, 1989.

Hagen-Ansert SL: Textbook of Diagnostic Ultrasonography, 3rd ed. St. Louis: C. V. Mosby, 1989.

Videos

The ability of static images to convey an appreciation of cardiac function is severely limited. Videos that demonstrate normal and abnormal cardiac states are almost essential for recognizing anything other than pericardial effusion and electromechanical dissociation.

Boswell R: Ultrasonography in Emergency Medicine Video Program, 301 University Blvd., Emergency Service—Route J73, Galveston, TX 77555-1073.

Gulfcoast Ultrasound: Introduction to adult echocardiography: vol. 1. P.O. Box 66700, St. Petersburg Beach, FL 33736.

Testicular Scanning Applications

Two of the most common cliches that medical students encounter in their first clinical year describe physician's tools (e.g., stethoscope, otoscope) as "an extension of the physician's own senses" and most every diagnostic or therapeutic procedure is deemed to be a "useful adjunct." Hackneyed though they may be, these two phrases properly describe the current role of ultrasound in the emergency department diagnosis of testicular and scrotal disease. There are relatively few conditions that present to the emergency department as acute testicular or scrotal problems. The diagnosis of these conditions has always relied primarily on the clinician's history and physical examination. In the past decade, a number of studies have emerged as adjuncts to the careful history of physical examination in sorting out scrotal disorders; ultrasound is one of these. Like technetium radionuclide scanning, hand-held audio Doppler, and transillumination, ultrasound can often be helpful in providing information regarding characteristics of the scrotal structure. But the information is ordinarily adjunctive in the true

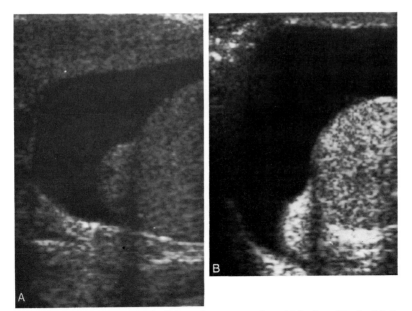

Figure 3–90. *A* and *B*. Normal testicle. These sagittal views demonstrate the epididymis and the testicle in patients with large hydroceles. The epididymis is usually of similar or slightly increased echogenicity to the normal testicle.

dence of inhomogeneity within the testicle itself. In the absence of an intercurrent spermatocele, no cystic structure is identified. More often than not, the ultrasound confirms the clinical impression of a normal testes and an inflamed epididymis. It certainly gives the clinician some reassurance as to the absence of testicular tumors, abscesses, or hydrocele. But if the initial concern was a distinction of epididymitis from torsion of the testes that could not be distinguished on clinical grounds, it is unlikely that the ultrasound alone (without Doppler) would be definitive in this differential.

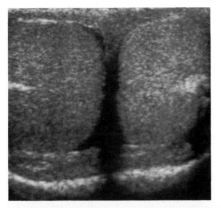

Figure 3–91. Mediastinum testis. The bright echogenic region seen in transverse scan represents the mediastinum testes (9 o'clock for right testicle; 3 o'clock for left testicle). This is the area where the tunica albuginea invaginates and the ducts and vessels enter into the testicle.

TORSION

The much-feared urologic emergency of torsion results from a twisting of the spermatic cord, which classically causes severe acute pain and in a matter of hours causes necrosis due to compromised arterial blood flow. In the typical case, the torsion causes the testicle to assume an unnatural, more horizontal position and, in the classic case, there should be absent blood flow demonstrable on color-flow Doppler or technetium scanning (Fig. 3–93*A* and *B*). Many cases, however, do not present classically and occur after several episodes of incomplete torsion, which may mimic epididymitis. Several findings have been described on ultrasound, including an enlarged, inhomogeneous testicular body and an enlarged epididymis, presumably the result of ischemia. The problem with such findings is that they are relatively late; by the time inhomogeneity is noted, ischemia is well established. Once again, standard ultrasound (without Doppler) is unlikely to be conclusive when the clinical examination and history are not.

There is a justifiable tendency to proceed with early surgical exploration for classic presentations of torsion if there is a high likelihood of this diagnosis. The use of color Doppler ultrasound for the early diagnosis of torsion gives flow information in addition to anatomic detail.

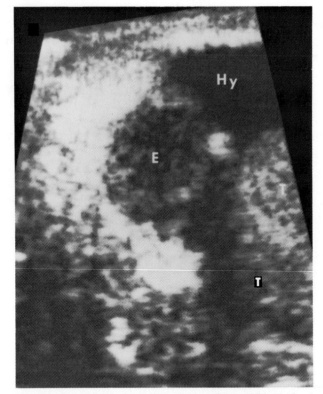

Figure 3–92. Acute epididymitis. This demonstrates the increase in size of the epididymis that is seen with both acute and chronic epididymitis. The epididymis (E) appears hypoechoic in comparison to the neighboring testicle (T) and is associated with a small reactive hydrocele (Hy). With chronic epididymitis, the epididymis may demonstrate focal echogenicities that represent calcifications. (From Sarti D: Ultrasonography of the scrotum. In Sarti D (ed): Diagnostic Ultrasound, 2nd ed. Chicago: Year Book Medical, 1987:589.)

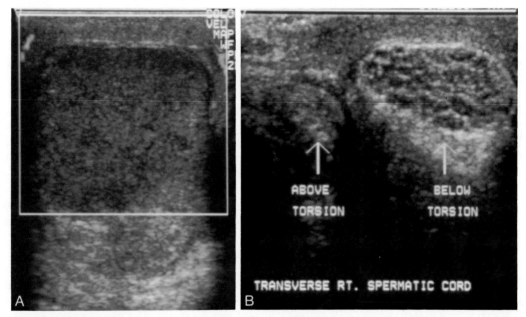

Figure 3–93. Testicular torsion. *A,* Demonstrates an image from a patient with testicular torsion. When the color-flow Doppler was turned on, there was no flow to this testicle. *B,* Demonstrates the appearance of the spermatic cord both above and below the level of torsion. There is significant dilation of the ducts and the venous structures below the torsion of the spermatic cord.

At the current time, experience with this technique varies widely among different institutions. Color-flow imaging can generally be helpful in ruling out torsion. Radionuclide scanning is used significantly in some institutions and hardly at all in others; the time required to obtain the study is clearly a major disadvantage, and interpretation of abnormalities requires considerable experience.

OTHER SCROTAL DISORDERS

Torsion of Testicular Appendages

The appendix epididymis and the appendix testis (Fig. 3–94) are two small, residual structures that can create major diagnostic problems for emergency physicians. When either of these structures undergoes torsion, the patient may present with acute testicular pain but without the associated physical signs one would expect with torsion of the testes themselves. The diagnosis is fairly often suspected but nonoperative diagnosis has been difficult. Transillumination (the blue dot sign) and radionuclide scanning are rarely diagnostic; ultrasound may demonstrate a tender, cystic structure in the appropriate region.

Hydrocele

Hydrocele is a collection of fluid between two layers of the tunica vaginalis that is easily visualized by ultrasound. As Figure 3–95A and B

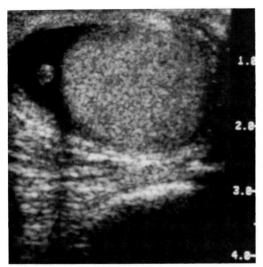

Figure 3–94. Appendix testis. This small appendage is an embryonic remnant, usually found near the head of the epididymis.

demonstrates, the testicle itself is normal and usually well visualized due to the acoustic window provided by the hydrocele.

Testicular Abscess

Although not very common, testicular abscess may form within the body of the testis, usually as a result of gonococcal infection. Affected patients are often febrile, have severe scrotal pain, and have evidence of a recent urethral discharge. Demonstration of an intratesticular abscess is easily accomplished by ultrasound and mandates urologic consultation and usually admission and drainage.

Other Testicular Problems

From the standpoint of the emergency physician, any significant area of inhomogeneity of the testicle should be recognized as abnormal and cause for referral. Unlike the epididymis, where malignancy is virtually unknown, masses of the testicle are frequently malignant.

Testicular Trauma

The emergency use of ultrasound for testicular scanning may be most helpful in the traumatized testicle. As might be expected, the testicle can fracture with surrounding hemorrhage, or the bleeding may be maintained within the capsule of the testicle, giving rise to a subcapsular hematoma. Ultrasound is considered the procedure of choice in diagnosing this condition (Fig. 3–96).

Varicoceles, Spermatoceles, Epididymal Cyst

Although varioceles, spermatoceles, and epididymal cysts are embryologically and anatomically distinct, they have much in common both clinically and in terms of their ultrasound appearances. All appear in sonographic cross sections to be cystic structures (i.e., black, echo-free interior surrounded by a more reflective wall) that are distinct from the body of the testicle (Figs. 3–97 to 3–99). The varicocele actually represents dilatation of the veins of the pampiniform plexus of the spermatic cord. These tubular venous structures occur more commonly on the left than the right.

All three structures are sometimes found on examination of the emergency patient who presents with scrotal pain and tenderness. Often, palpation reveals some tenderness, but

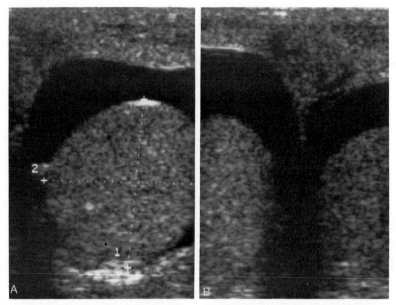

Figure 3–95. Hydroceles. These images illustrate the appearance of unilateral (*A*) and bilateral (*B*) hydroceles. Note the improved visualization of the testicle secondary to the window provided by the fluid collection.

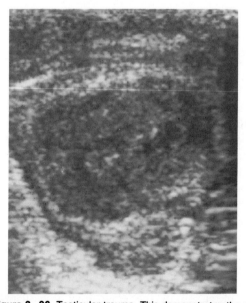

Figure 3–96. Testicular trauma. This demonstrates the ultrasound appearance of a testicular contusion. Note the inhomogeneous echoes in the parenchyma of the testicle.

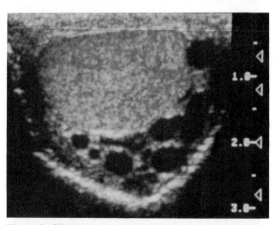

Figure 3–97. Varicocele. Note the dilated venous structures in the lower portion of the image adjacent to the testicle. This represents dilation of the pampiniform plexus. Varicoceles occur more commonly on the left side than on the right.

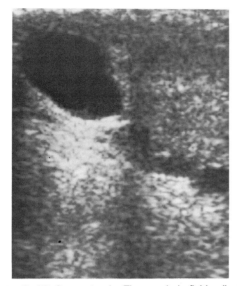

Figure 3-98. Spermatocele. The anechoic fluid collection superior to the testicle proved to be a spermatocele.

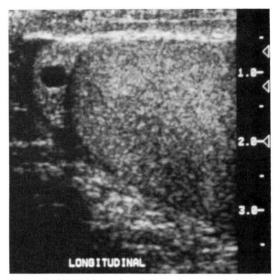

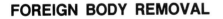

Figure 3-99. Epididymal cyst. There is an anechoic structure within the head of the epididymis, representing an epididymal cyst.

the precise mechanisms of pain and its relationship to these benign conditions are often unclear.

SELECTED READINGS

Testicular Scanning Applications

Benson CB, Doubilet PM, Richie JP: Sonography of the male genital tract. AJR 1989;153:705–713.
Benson CB, Doubilet PM, Vickers MA: Sonography of the penis. Ultrasound Q 1991;9:89–109.
Fowler RC, Chennells PM, Ewing R: Scrotal ultrasonography: A clinical evaluation. Br J Radiol 1987;60:649–654.

Hill MC, Sanders RC: Sonography of benign disease of the scrotum. Ultrasound Annual 1986;197–237.

Texts

Virtually all the general texts have sections dealing with scrotal ultrasound, which includes torsion, epididymis, and trauma.

Goldberg's Textbook of Abdominal Ultrasound. Baltimore: Williams & Wilkins, 1993. *The most complete and recent, with a useful discussion of penile disorders and trauma as well.*
Mittelstaedt's Abdominal Ultrasound. New York: Churchill Livingstone, 1992. *Also bears mention.*

Procedural Applications

FOREIGN BODY REMOVAL

Foreign bodies may not seem like the most important problem in emergency medicine, but they are a source of much frustration, considerable expenditure of time and energy, and many lawsuits. In fact, failure to remove foreign bodies from wounds prior to closure is said to represent the second most common cause of malpractice suits against emergency physicians. There are three separate aspects to the problem. First is the issue of ensuring that any given laceration or even any puncture wound does not harbor an unsuspected foreign body. Second is the problem of the patient presenting to the emergency department with clear evidence (often infection or failure to heal a wound) of a foreign body. Third is the technical question of how to best remove a foreign body when its presence is known. Emergency department ultrasound may be helpful in all three situations.

Sonographic Considerations

Foreign bodies may be made of almost any material; some of the most common ones are not visualized by standard radiographic examination. Although glass, metal, and gravel are examples of familiar materials that are well visualized by radiographs, wood, thorns, and some plastics are almost entirely radiolucent. Recent studies have examined the ability of ultrasound to detect such substances using a variety of models. Because most foreign bodies in the emergency department are both small and superficial, a high-resolution, 7.5-MHz transducer is used.

It appears that ultrasound is capable of detecting foreign bodies composed of any of these materials down to the size of approximately 1 to 2 mm. Unfortunately, most studies employ the technique of embedding foreign bodies in meat or chicken wings. Clinical studies in emergency department patients are sorely needed. Used prophylactically on a high-risk laceration prior to closure, sterile gel is applied to the wound and a sterile condom or rubber examination glove is fitted over the transducer head. Scanning is performed in at least two planes, extending beyond the laceration at least several centimeters in each direction. All foreign bodies appear as hyperechoic foci; some cause shadowing, others have a "comet-tail" that represents reverberation artifact (Fig. 3–100). Hard copy can be generated to document the ultrasound appearance of the wound prior to closure.

Clinical Considerations

The first problem facing the emergency physician is to define upon presentation what wounds require more than the usual search and irrigation prior to closure. For many, if not most wounds, the mechanism of injury and appearance of the lesion practically rule out the presence of a foreign body. With appropriate documentation of that history, no imaging procedure would be indicated. Conversely, there are some high-risk wounds, in terms of mechanism of injury or appearance of the wound, in which the likelihood of a foreign body clearly justifies an imaging procedure (even if not infallible) for the preclosure identification of foreign bodies. A sizable number of wounds come between these two extremes, in which the risk seems moderate but not negligible. No clear standard of care has been defined for this group, but there is growing support for an aggressive approach that uses both x-ray and ultrasound where appropriate for virtually all such patients. It appears likely, but is not proven, that the addition of ultrasound examination will improve the emergency physician's ability to identify foreign bodies.

Some element of clinical judgment is still necessary in determining what does and does not constitute a low-risk wound, but some guidelines can be promulgated although they have not been rigorously studied. These criteria are summarized in Table 3–3; a wound is not considered low risk if any of the criteria listed there apply.

The type of imaging procedure to be used is then determined on the basis of the known etiologic properties of the suspected foreign bodies involved. If the history is clear as to the composition of the suspected foreign bodies, either

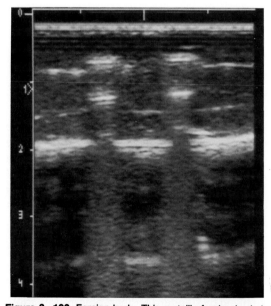

Figure 3–100. Foreign body. This metallic foreign body is echogenic and demonstrates "comet-tail" shadowing. Two segments of the foreign body are seen in this view.

Table 3–3. CRITERIA FOR DETERMINING WOUND RISK

1. Reported mechanism of injury associated with foreign body deposition; the appearance of the wound indicates a possibility of foreign body
2. The appearance of the wound is not consistent with the history obtained
3. A reliable history is not available, regardless of what the wound looks like
4. Any foreign body is seen in the wound
5. Any foreign body was previously removed from the wound prior to arriving in the emergency department
6. The patient is concerned that there might be a foreign body in the wound, regardless of history and appearance

x-ray, ultrasound, or a combination of both may be utilized. In cases where the wound is truly high risk by traditional criteria, both x-ray and ultrasound should be used unless the foreign bodies are highly radiopaque (i.e., metal). In the absence of clinical studies directly comparing the accuracy of the two imaging techniques, this type of course seems justified. In addition, ultrasound localization of foreign bodies, like all ultrasound imaging, is a user-dependent skill that almost certainly improves with experience. Using a plan such as that outlined ensures that the physician will not only gain experience in the technique, but also have at least some basis for comparison with the traditional practice of standard radiology.

Finally, the question of how to remove a foreign body once it has been found by radiograph or ultrasound has no single answer. Many superficial foreign bodies can be rapidly palpated with a gloved finger or an instrument and removed without difficulty. For foreign bodies that cannot be palpated, using real-time ultrasound for guidance has many advantages over the blind method. It is also far more rapid and inexpensive than the well-known method of skin markers and repeated plain radiographs to localize the foreign body in relation to the skin marker. After administering appropriate local anesthesia, the wound is covered with sterile gel extending 2 cm beyond the wound edge in the region where the foreign body may be localized. Using as small an instrument as possible, appropriate to the size of the foreign body (e.g., a mosquito clamp for an object several millimeters in diameter), the transducer is placed in the nondominant hand on the intact gelled surface of the skin, between 1 and 2 cm from the wound edge. The physician angles the ultrasound beam so that the foreign body image is projected in the middle of the field. The instrument is then directed toward the location of the foreign body, and the ultrasound appearance of the instrument (which is less distinct than might be expected) is confirmed by its movement. The foreign body is then grasped and removed.

Application of emergency department ultrasound to the problem of foreign bodies has occurred just as significant deficiencies in the emergency department approach to foreign bodies has been acknowledged. It is not possible to state how our standards for the management of this common clinical problem will evolve, but

it is likely that emergency department ultrasound will have a role.

SUPRAPUBIC ASPIRATION

Suprapubic aspiration of the urinary bladder to obtain urine is a commonly performed procedure in infants in the course of doing a septic work-up. Much has been written concerning the relative safety of the technique, particularly as compared to Foley catheterization, but the incidence of "dry taps" is reported to be in the 50% range. Two or three aspirations are attempted; if they are unsuccessful, the bladder is assumed to be empty and the child is given time to fill his or her bladder in order to void spontaneously for the specimen. Clearly, the use of bedside ultrasound to localize the bladder first and ascertain that urine is present would be suspected to greatly increase the effects of this procedure. A recent study that used ultrasound as a localizing device (not as a guide during the aspiration itself) demonstrated just that. A pediatric intensive care unit, using ultrasound guidance during the puncture, reported a success rate of 100%. If bedside ultrasound is available in the department, it should be used prior to suprapubic aspiration.

GYNECOLOGIC PROCEDURES

Sonographic Guidance of Clinical Procedures

There are two emergent gynecologic procedures in which diagnostic ultrasound can be of significant benefit: culdocentesis and suction curettage.

Culdocentesis

Although the increasing availability of diagnostic ultrasound and sensitive urine and serum hormone testing has almost obviated the need for culdocentesis in many institutions, there remain certain clinical situations where the procedure is useful. For example, the ultrasound finding of significant pelvic fluid in a patient with severe abdominal pain may raise the issue of ruptured ovarian cyst versus ruptured ectopic pregnancy. In some cases, the differentiation between the two may depend on the quality of the fluid that is aspirated from the culdocentesis. The hemoperitoneum seen from ruptured ectopic pregnancy is ordinarily distinguished

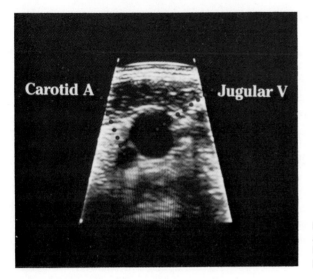

Figure 3 – 101. Vascular access. The internal jugular vein and carotid artery are seen in this view. The internal jugular is located more laterally and is compressible with the probe.

from the thinner, more serous fluid of a ruptured ovarian cyst. Although it is traditionally done in a blind fashion, culdocentesis can be facilitated by visualizing the fluid pocket transabdominally while the aspirating needle is advanced into the cul-de-sac. A 20- or 21-gauge spinal needle usually can be clearly seen sonographically as it enters the fluid-filled pouch.

Suction Curettage

Although suction curettage of incomplete spontaneous abortions is now commonly performed as an outpatient procedure, it is not usually performed by emergency physicians except in truly emergency settings or when a specialty consultation is not available. Transabdominal ultrasound scanning performed simultaneously with suction curettage has the advantage of identifying the fundus of the uterus, the character and volume of the remaining uterine content, and the curettage catheter. Thus, the risk of uterine perforation is decreased.

VASCULAR ACCESS

It would seem obvious that ultrasound guidance would improve the success and safety of central venous (and arterial) access. Using the high-resolution transducer, commonly accessed vessels such as the internal jugular and femoral veins are well visualized. Standard needles can be visualized by the artifact they produce. In addition, specialized equipment, such

as needle guides and highly reflective needles (used for sonographically guided biopsies) are well suited for vascular access.

Thus far, however, there have only been a few brief reports of such use in the emergency department, perhaps reflecting the relative scarcity of appropriate equipment in emergency departments or perhaps a feeling of confidence that the traditional blind approach is satisfactory. Very impressive reports from the cardiology literature have documented that ultrasound guidance can decrease the number of attempts required for central line insertion and alert the physician to anatomic conditions that would make cannulation dangerous or impossible. Using a non-Doppler unit and a 7.5-MHz transducer with a needle holder, the internal jugular and carotid vessels are visualized (Fig. 3 – 101) and a Valsalva maneuver is performed that distends the jugular vein prior to the guided puncture. Cannulation then proceeds in the usual manner. This cannulation technique appears to be very valuable in those patients where intravenous access is known or expected to be challenging.

SELECTED READINGS

Procedural Applications

Banerjee B, Das RK: Sonographic detection of foreign bodies of the extremities. Br J Radiol 1991;64:107–112.

Crawford R, Matheson AB: Clinical value of ultrasonography in the detection and removal of radiolucent foreign bodies. Injury 1989;20:341–343.

Denys BG, Uretsky BF, Reddy SJ, et al: An ultrasound

method for safe and rapid central venous access. N Engl J Med 1991;324(8):566.

Fornage BD, Schernberg FL: Sonographic diagnosis of foreign bodies of the distal extremities. AJR 1986;147:567–569.

Gilbert FJ, Campbell RSD, Bayliss AP: The role of ultrasound in the detection of non-radiopaque foreign bodies. Clin Radiol 1990;41:109–112.

Gochman RF, Karasic RB, Heller MB: Use of portable ultrasound to assist urine collection by suprapubic aspiration. Ann Emerg Med 1991;20:631–635.

Koski EM, Suhonen M, Mattila MA: Ultrasound-facilitated central venous cannulation. Crit Care Med 1992; 20(3):424–426.

O'Callaghan C, McDougall PN: Successful suprapubic aspiration of urine. Arch Dis Child 1987;62:1072–1073.

Schlager D, Sanders AB, Wiggins D, et al: Ultrasound for the detection of foreign bodies. Ann Emerg Med 1991; 20:189–191.

Equipment Criteria

An impressive variety of ultrasound equipment is available. Fortunately, by combining a basic knowledge of ultrasound instrumentation (see Chapter 1) with a clear knowledge of the planned applications of ultrasound in a particular emergency department, it is possible to rationally limit the options to a small number of choices that then can be compared and selected on the basis of personal preference. The goal of this section is simply to present and discuss the considerations that might form part of that process.

MINIMUM REQUIREMENTS

There are certain minimum criteria that are so basic for emergency department ultrasound that they should be mandatory in any proposed system.

Adequate Image Quality. There are several technical ways to measure image quality. For clinical purposes, only two bear mention. First, the scanner should be capable of displaying the image in at least 64 shades of gray; any less than this will significantly compromise identification and will certainly impair the quality of the hard copy produced. Secondly, there should be an adequate screen size of at least 5 inches diagonally. Although screen size itself does not determine resolution or image quality, scanners with very small (2- to 3-inch) screens are impractical for routine emergency department use and often require placing the device physically on the patient or in an awkward position. They also virtually prevent the patient from viewing the ultrasound examination and it is difficult for

more than one physician to see the screen as well.

Measurement Capabilities. Many ultrasound distinctions between normal and abnormal are quantitative. The diameter of the aorta and thickness of the gallbladder and of the common duct are but a few examples. It is therefore necessary that the equipment include, at a minimum, an on-screen caliper system that allows for measurement at least of one length with simultaneous display of that measurement on screen.

Freeze Frame. Many events observed in emergency real-time scanning are observed only fleetingly. In order to appreciate them best, show them to others, as well as to record them on hard copy, it is necessary that a simple system for freezing the frame is integrated into the device.

Permanent Record Making (Hard Copy). There are times in the emergency use of ultrasound that hard copy is not required, such as determination of fetal demise, documentation of electromechanical dissociation, and when the technique is used as an aid to perform some clinical procedures. Indeed, there are times when ultrasound is used as a stethoscope, as part of a screening examination, as a teaching tool, or in those situations where the results of the examination have little clinical import that the generation of hard copy is unnecessary. However, when the examination is done in a more formal manner, as is usually true in investigation of the chief complaint, and when results of the examination are of clinical significance, it is mandatory that hard copy images be generated. In addition, hard copy is required for maintenance of a quality assurance program and, by regulation, if a professional bill is generated. Several adequate hard copy systems exist. Most systems that generate images on film, akin to those used in computed tomography, are associated with more expensive ultrasound devices and are not yet common in emergency departments. The most often used system is a free-standing printer that prints the screen image on specially treated paper. The graphic systems that require taking an actual photograph of the screen rather than electronic transfer of screen contents are unsuitable for routine use.

Mobility Appropriate to the Facility. Emergency ultrasound is used for such an eclectic group of patients that it is not ordinarily feasible to confine these patients all to a single room or space. The device must therefore be capable of being moved easily, ordinarily on a small, wheeled cart, and of fitting into the often cramped examining rooms that comprise many emergency departments. All the accessories necessary — transducers, gel, hard copy printer, etc. — should fit comfortably on this cart as well.

This short list should be viewed as a minimum. There are only a few devices produced today that do not fill these criteria; many older units could fulfill them as well.

DESIRABLE FEATURES

As the emergency department use of ultrasound is in a state of rapid evaluation, the patterns of use vary greatly. In some departments, for example, ultrasound use is reserved for only gynecologic problems; in others, the main use is cardiac. Desirability of any particular feature would clearly vary greatly at these two extremes. In most institutions, however, ultrasound is being used or will be used for the basic emergency department indications discussed in this book. It is therefore almost always prudent to at least allow for the possibility of these standard uses in the selection of a device that either possesses capabilities for the major emergency department indications or that can be upgraded.

Sector Scanning. Although linear array scanning has been widely used for most of the indications applicable to emergency medicine, it is clear that the capacity for sector scanning is very desirable. The greater flexibility afforded by sector scanning in proximity to the thorax is highly desirable. Some devices have the capability for multiple types of transducers, which is an advantage that allows the physician to choose which transducer is best for the particular patient and the particular area being studied. The curved array transducer is an increasingly popular option that combines many of the advantages of sector and linear scanning. The ability to magnify or diminish the size of the field on the screen is also important. In addition, the more sophisticated systems have zoom magnification features.

Variable Focal Length. It may be recalled that the focal length is the distance from the transducer head, where the ultrasound beam is most compacted. It is at this precise spot that the most optimal images are produced and some artifacts are avoided. Because it is not always possible to place the area of interest at the focal length, it is desirable that there should be some means available for altering this. Two distinct focal lengths, a near and a far field, are probably adequate. The same effect can be achieved by using transducers with different focal lengths.

Adequate Compatible Transducer Capability. This is the most difficult and most important feature in this category. Ultrasound machines vary considerably in this capability, and the requirements of individual emergency departments vary as well. At least 3.5- and 5-MHz transducers should be available in the emergency department. The lower frequency transducer head should be shaped appropriately for intercostal scanning.

A high-resolution (7.5-MHz) transducer, although not necessary for the major emergency department applications, is absolutely necessary if ultrasound is to be used for foreign body localization or scanning blood vessels; it is also very desirable for testicular scanning and suprapubic aspiration in infants. It is feasible (but may not be optimal) to use specialized transducers (e.g., endovaginal) for other functions if their frequency and focal lengths are appropriate.

Endovaginal Transducer Capabilities. Unless the institution's practices and policies are such that transvaginal scanning is never performed in the emergency department, the undisputed advantages of this approach for the diagnosis of early ectopic pregnancy make this mandatory. Both the standard of care and local practices are evolving so quickly in this area that a transvaginal transducer should be available for a particular instrument, even if it is not used initially.

OTHER ULTRASOUND OPTIONS

There are several other ultrasound features that are useful but that may be of only marginal value in the emergency department.

Doppler Ultrasound. The addition of ultrasound to Doppler, either scaler or color Doppler, allows for the determination of flow information at the same time that anatomic information is displayed on the image. A powerful and still somewhat expensive tool, it is not required for any of the major emergency indications, but would be helpful in many applications by making it much easier to identify vascular structures. For cardiac, vascular, and aortic scanning, the advantages are evident, and Doppler aids the distinction between torsion and epididymitis of the painful testicle. The cost of additional Doppler capabilities has been decreasing steadily over the last few years. It is likely that Doppler will be a common feature in emergency ultrasound over the next 5 to 10 years.

Videotaping Capability. Most but not all ultrasound monitors allow the user to videotape the examination by using a standard videocassette recorder (VCR). Some offer this as a built-in capability. This feature might be especially desirable in institutions where tapes of the actual examinations are used for teaching purposes and will be necessary in those institutions where quality assurance programs mandate the review of the real-time examinations.

Internal Memory. Some ultrasound devices allow the frozen image to be stored in memory, where it can be reviewed later or printed out as hard copy. This may actually facilitate the examination, because multiple images can be stored electronically without having to pause for the generation of hard copies. The stored images can be recalled later and only the best ones printed as hard copy; this has advantages for teaching as well.

Internal Software. Many devices include software packages that provide such useful data as crown–rump length and normal values for sizes of various organs. This is perhaps less important for emergency applications than for more specialized uses, but a program that generates estimated dates of confinement and fetal age based on various fetal measurements is helpful. Some units have software that allows the user to program it with whatever information is believed to be useful. This would allow immediate access to such data as normal gallbladder wall thickness and duct sizes.

Image Labeling. Almost all newer devices have the capability to print identifying information on the image itself. These are most commonly letters or words used to identify various structures; they appear on the ultrasound screen and are reproduced on the hard copy with patient/user information printed under the image. Some devices include an icon that represents the patient in various anatomic positions and allows the user to place body markers in the appropriate location, indicating the orientation of the transducer head when the image was taken.

Foot Pedal Control (Remote Controls). Most machines offer the option of using a foot pedal control to start and stop scanning. In emergency departments, where the ultrasound device is moved frequently from room to room, this is unlikely to be used consistently.

Variable Frequency Transducers. Several devices are marketed that combine two or three transducer frequencies in the same hand-held unit, with the option of switching from one frequency to the next merely by pushing a button. This is a minor convenience in emergency medicine and, like the foot pedal, is more appropriate for use in ultrasound laboratories.

Split Screen. In this option, the ultrasound screen is split in half and two images are developed. This allows for convenient depiction of both before and after images. This is used for demonstrating the effects of various maneuvers (pressure, Valsalva) and has little direct emergency department application.

M-Mode. Many devices allow for scanning in M-mode. This allows for hard-copy documentation of the presence or absence of the fetal heartbeat.

Transesophageal Echo (TEE) Capability. Although not now used by emergency physicians, the technique of transesophageal echocardiography is being used more and more frequently by cardiologists in investigation of chest pain and suspected thoracic aortic dissection. In many places, it is now the procedure of choice for diagnosing this condition, which often cannot be excluded by surface echocardiography.

Cost Considerations. Unlike most everything else, the past few years have seen a reduction in the cost of ultrasound devices, particularly the entry-level units that are suitable for most emergency department needs. Several manufacturers now offer ultrasound devices that include all the mandatory features noted above as well as two transducers for no more than $25,000. Additional transducers often cost $7000 to $9000; Doppler capabilities vary by manufacturer, but would generally require at least another $10,000.

Model Curriculum for Physician Training in Emergency Ultrasonography

There is a growing interest in the bedside use of ultrasonography by emergency physicians. Research has demonstrated the utility of these techniques in the emergency department setting.[1-9] It is apparent that bedside ultrasonography is a very helpful adjunct for the diagnosis of a number of emergent and life-threatening conditions.

As emergency physicians have begun to apply this technology, questions have developed regarding appropriate utilization, training, and credentialing. In response to this, the American College of Emergency Physicians published a position statement on ultrasound in 1990, stating that emergency ultrasonography should be performed by appropriately trained and credentialed physicians, including emergency physicians.[10] The Society for Academic Emergency Medicine (SAEM) endorsed this position, and in addition recommended that a curriculum and training objectives be developed for emergency medicine programs that elect to

Reproduced from Mateer J, Plummer D, Heller M, Olson D, Jehle D, Overton D, Gussow L: Model curriculum for physician training in emergency ultrasonography. Ann Emerg Med 1994;23:95–102. With permission from Mosby-Year Book, Inc.

train their residents in ultrasonography, and for practicing emergency physicians who seek postgraduate training in this area.[11]

The purpose of this document is to define an ultrasonography curriculum that may be incorporated into emergency medicine residency programs, and to recommend criteria for training of practicing physicians in emergency ultrasonography.

METHODS

The SAEM Ultrasound Task Force is comprised of academic emergency physicians who currently use ultrasonography and are training emergency medicine residents and practicing emergency physicians in ultrasonography techniques. A problem-oriented outline of educational objectives was created by selecting topics and conditions that meet one or more of the following criteria:

1. A life-threatening or serious medical condition

2. A condition in which ultrasonography is accepted as a primary diagnostic modality

3. A condition in which an ultrasound exami-

nation would significantly decrease costs or time associated with patient evaluation

4. A situation where ultrasonography serves as an adjunct for a commonly performed emergency procedure

5. Essential background material for those who perform or interpret diagnostic ultrasound examinations

Standard textbooks, education videos, and articles were referenced so that an adequate working library could be acquired. The average number of hours of didactic, reading, and case review needed to adequately study the material was suggested for each section. The material was divided into four primary sections (physics, cardiovascular, abdominal, and OB/GYN) and one optional section on additional uses. The additional uses section was included to identify material that may be useful for emergency physicians when the interest, clinical material, and educational commitment exists within a program. Specific educational methods and time for this section were not suggested, because programs may elect to use only portions of this additional material. The average minimum number of training examinations needed to learn basic emergency ultrasound techniques was determined based on the experience of the Task Force members. These minimums were established to define the criterion for completion of initial training, and although it is helpful to perform initial examinations in normal models, it is intended that at least 50% of these training examinations would consist of clinically indicated patient studies. It is understood that, as with any diagnostic imaging technique, confidence continues to develop as the interpreting physician becomes more experienced.

PHYSICS AND INSTRUMENTATION*

A. General wave physics
  1. Wave character (12:10–17)
     a. Cycle
     b. Frequency
     c. Period
     d. Wavelength
     e. Amplitude
     f. Speed

*Numbers in parentheses refer to references at the end of this curriculum. Numbers following the colon, if any, refer to specific pages within the book or article referenced.

2. Pulsed ultrasound (12:20–25)
   a. Pulse frequency
   b. Pulse duration
   c. Spacial pulse length
   d. Duty factor
3. Attenuation (12:28–38)
   a. Intensity
   b. Frequency vs. depth
4. Tissue interaction (12:41–51)
   a. Reflection, echoes
   b. Transmission
   c. Scatter
5. Bioeffects (12:219–225)
   a. Thermal
   b. Cavitation
6. Safety (12:226–229)
B. Instrumentation
   1. Transducers (12:66–73)
      a. Pulse generation
         (1) Piezoelectric effect
         (2) Continuous beam
         (3) Pulsed beam
         (4) Bandwidth
   2. Beam Focusing (12:74–81)
      a. Beam diameter
         (1) Unfocused beam
            a) Near zone
            b) Far zone
         (2) Focused beam
   3. Probe types (12:83–87; 13:1–14)
      a. Linear array
      b. Mechanical sector
      c. Phased array
      d. Annular array
   4. Resolution (12:89–99)
      a. Axial
      b. Lateral
   5. Receiver controls (12:110–117)
      a. Gain
      b. Compensation (TGC)
      c. Rejection
   6. Imaging modes (12:130–137)
      a. A-mode
      b. B-mode
      c. M-mode
      d. B scan (2-D)
   7. Imaging artifacts (12:147–173)
      a. Reverberation
      b. Refraction
      c. Mirror image
      d. Shadowing
      e. Enhancement
      f. Comet tail

g. Ring-down
C. Suggested educational methods
1. Lecture (1 hour) and/or
2. Structured reading program (2–4 hours) and/or
3. Physics video (1 hour) (14) and/or
4. Interactive computer program (15)

CARDIOVASCULAR

A. Anatomy (16:73–101)
1. Cardiac chambers
2. Cardiac valves
3. Endocardium
4. Myocardium
5. Pericardium
6. Papillary muscles
7. Great vessels
B. Techniques/equipment (16:50–51; 17)
1. Standard windows
a. Left parasternal
1) Long axis
2) Short axis
b. Apical
c. Subcostal
2. Transducer selection
C. Pericardial fluid (16:548–558; 18)
1. Definition
2. Etiologies (16:565–567)
3. Echocardiographic features
D. Cardiac tamponade (16:588–565; 18; 19)
1. Definition
2. Echocardiographic features
3. Sensitivity/specificity
E. Acute chest pain (6; 16; 20) Differential diagnosis
1. Cardiac ischemia
2. Pulmonary embolism (21)
3. Pericarditis (22)
4. Aortic dissection
F. Ischemic complications (16:482–495; 23)
1. Pump failure
2. Effusion (24)
3. Ventricular septal defect
4. Papillary muscle dysfunction
5. Left ventricular thrombus
6. Aneurysm formation
7. Myocardial rupture
G. Hypotension/dyspnea (16; 21; 22)
1. Classification
2. Echocardiographic features
a. Hypovolemic
b. Cardiogenic

c. Acute outflow obstruction
d. Acute inflow obstruction
H. Cardiac arrest—EMD (3)
1. Cardiogenic
2. Noncardiogenic (4)
I. Trauma
1. Penetrating (2)
a. Hemopericardium
2. Blunt (25)
a. Cardiac contusion
b. Cardiac rupture
J. Suggested educational methods
1. Lecture (2–3 hours) and/or
2. Structured reading program (3–6 hours)
3. Case reviews (2–4 hours)
4. Technical skills—minimum 50 cardiac examinations (including standard windows)

ABDOMINAL

A. Anatomy (26:198–300)
1. Gallbladder
a. Normal size
b. Wall thickness
c. Common variants
2. Kidneys
a. Morison's pouch
b. Cortex
c. Pyramids
d. Sinus
e. Congenital variants (13:434–437, 454–460)
3. Aorta
a. Normal size
b. Major branches
4. Liver
5. Diaphragm
6. Spleen
7. Pancreas
8. Bowel
9. Other major vessels
B. Techniques/Equipment (27:7–19, 26–33)
1. Transducer options
a. Frequency
b. Sector vs. others
2. Techniques
a. Patient preparation
b. Scan planes
c. Orientation
C. Abdominal aortic aneurysm (13:402–408; 28:279–281; 7; 29)
1. Definition

2. Appearance
3. Extent/size
4. Thrombus/leakage
D. Biliary colic (26:225–245; 28:54–62; 30)
1. Cholelithiasis
a. Appearance
b. Shadowing
c. Dependency
d. Impaction
e. Ductal stones
2. Cholecystitis
a. Wall thickness
b. Tenderness
c. Gangrenous gallbladder
d. Emphysematous
e. Perforation
f. Pericholecystic fluid
3. Other Abnormalities
a. Sludge
b. Ductal dilatation (28:64–68)
c. Polyps/masses
d. Acalculous cholecystitis (28:62–64)
E. Renal colic (13:442–445, 486; 27:156–157; 31)
1. Hydronephrosis
a. Acute
b. Chronic
c. Bilateral
d. Significance (32:243–244)
2. Hydroureter
3. Calculi
F. Abdominal trauma (8,33)
1. Hemoperitoneum—locations
a. Hepatorenal recess (Morison's pouch)
b. Splenorenal recess
c. Paracolic gutters
d. Cul-de-sac
e. Retroperitoneal
f. Subdiaphragmatic
2. Organ injuries (32:78, 98–101, 230–232; 34) liver/spleen/kidneys
a. Intraparenchymal hematoma
b. Subcapsular hematoma
c. Fracture
d. Sensitivity/specificity
G. Suggested educational methods
1. Lecture (2–3 hours) and/or
2. Structured reading program (3–6 hours)
3. Case reviews (2–4 hours)
4. Technical skills—minimum 50 abdominal examinations (including above anatomy as appropriate)

OBSTETRIC AND GYNECOLOGIC

A. Anatomy (35:375–392)
1. Uterus/variants (35:394–403)
2. Endometrial stripe
3. Vagina
4. Cul-de-sac
5. Ovaries (35:424–426)
6. Bladder
7. Iliac vessels
8. Bowel
9. Muscles
B. Techniques/equipment
1. Transabdominal (26:409–413)
a. Equipment
b. Patient preparation
c. Scanning planes/procedure
2. Transvaginal
a. Equipment (36:29–37)
b. Patient/probe preparation (36:61–64)
c. Scanning planes/procedures (36:64–75)
d. Comparison of transabdominal and transvaginal (36:77–107)
C. Intrauterine pregnancy—first trimester (35:19–29)
1. Normal sonoembryology
a. Decidual reaction
b. Gestational sac
c. Double decidual sac
d. Yolk sac
e. Amnion
f. Fetal pole/embryo
g. Placenta
h. Cardiac activity
i. Corpus luteum cyst (35:44)
2. Gestational age (35:47–59, 29–31)
a. Sac size
b. Crown–rump length
c. Biparietal diameter
3. Documentation (35:3–4)
a. Location of IUP
b. Size/dates
c. Fetal number
d. Fetal heart rate
e. Abnormal findings
D. Ectopic pregnancy (35:447–466; 36:233–235)
1. Risk factors
2. Complementary tests
a. Serum hCG—discriminatory zone (36:233–235)

b. Serum progesterone (37, 38)
3. Decidual cast
4. Pseudogestational sac
5. Ectopic sac
6. Adnexal ring/mass
7. Cul-de-sac fluid
8. Heterotopic pregnancy
9. Interstitial pregnancy (39, 40)
10. Cervical pregnancy (41, 42)
11. Pitfalls (43)
E. Abortion (35:32–43; 36:299–325)
1. Threatened abortion
a. Prognostic factors
2. Incomplete abortion
a. Retained products (44)
3. Embryonic/fetal demise
a. Criteria for fetal death
4. Abembryonic pregnancy (blighted ovum)
F. Third trimester bleeding
1. Placenta previa (35:304–308; 36:211–219)
a. Migration
b. Imaging techniques
2. Abruption (35:308–315; 45:1611)
a. Limitations of ultrasound
b. Complementary tests
G. Trauma in pregnancy (45:1611)
1. Fetal viability
2. Gestational age
3. Limitations/complementary tests
4. Intraperitoneal hemorrhage
H. Suggested educational methods
1. Lecture (2–3 hours) and/or
2. Structured reading program (3–6 hours)
3. Case Reviews (2–4 hours)
4. Technical Skills—Minimum
a. Transabdominal—25 examinations
b. Transvaginal—25 examinations

ADDITIONAL USES/ISSUES (OPTIONAL)

Cardiovascular

A. Myocardial ischemia (46, 47, 48)
1. Left ventricle segmental mapping (16:462–468; 49)
2. Right ventricular infarction (16:495–497; 50)
3. Size of infarction (16:476–479)
B. Valvular disease (13:642–656)
1. Mitral valve

2. Aortic valve
3. Endocarditis (16:312–319; 18:196–202)
C. Advanced cardiovascular techniques
1. Doppler and color flow (12:177–199)
2. Transesophageal echocardiography (51, 52, 53)
D. Vascular
1. Deep vein thrombosis (32:668–673; 54)
a. Anatomy/techniques
b. Duplex imaging
c. Significance
2. Arterial (32:642–648)
a. Anatomy/techniques
b. Stenosis
c. Plaque hemorrhage/ulceration

Abdominal

E. Miscellaneous abdominal
1. Liver (32:51, 56–65, 75–77)
a. Hepatomegaly
b. Abscess
c. Metastasis
d. Cirrhosis/ascites
2. Pancreas (32:155–164)
a. Pancreatitis
b. Pseudocysts
3. Diaphragm (32:368–371, 377)
a. Pleural effusion/hemothorax (13:744–746)
4. Bowel (32:193–198)
a. Appendicitis (55, 56)
b. Bowel obstruction
5. Urinary tract (32:226–227, 216–225)
a. Renal infection/abscess
b. Renal cysts
c. Renal masses
d. Bladder residual volume

Obstetric and Gynecologic

F. Pelvic inflammatory disease (36:138–141; 57; 58)
1. Hydrosalpinx
2. Pyosalpinx
3. Tubo-ovarian complex
4. Pelvic abscess
G. Pelvic masses
1. Uterine masses (35:403–410)
2. Adnexal masses (35:429–446; 36:149–168)
a. Simple cyst
b. Complex cyst
c. Solid mass

Soft Tissues

Interventional Ultrasound

Administrative Issues

DISCUSSION

Although ultrasonography has been used in Europe at the bedside to assist in the diagnosis of acute conditions for many years, this concept has only been recently considered in the United States. A growing number of emergency physicians are using bedside ultrasonography to enhance their diagnostic accuracy and speed in the recognition of emergent and life-threatening conditions. Reports in the literature show that bedside use by clinicians improves patient care.[1-9]

Ultrasound imaging techniques and interpretation are not always straightforward, and there are pitfalls that must be recognized. The scope of ultrasound knowledge that applies to emergency medicine, however, is limited to conditions that present acutely or where results affect immediate patient management or disposition. The model curriculum described previously defines the training that emergency physicians need in order to begin using bedside emergency ultrasonography in this manner.

A number of emergency medicine programs have initiated ultrasonography training for their residents. When these residents complete their training, the program director is responsible for determining whether they are considered trained in emergency ultrasonography. Because the use of ultrasonography in emergency medicine is relatively new and has the potential of becoming a standard procedure for emergency medicine training in the future, we believe that guidelines should exist to assist a program director with this decision. The model curriculum has been developed by academic emergency physicians to recommend the content of basic ultrasonography training provided to residents. In this manner, the quality and accuracy of training in emergency medicine ultrasonography may be assured.

This model curriculum can be incorporated into current educational sessions of an emergency medicine residency program. Alternatively, the didactic portion, as well as some of the hands-on training, could occur during special seminars scheduled by the program director. The suggested didactic hours were determined based on a formal lecture presentation format. A program director may elect to provide some or all of this material through a structured reading program or other educational methods.

Case reviews that include ultrasound images are a powerful educational tool. Technical skills can be acquired through hands-on sessions with a sonographer or faculty. It is important for at least one emergency medicine faculty member to become skilled in ultrasonography in order to coordinate this program. Initial training ultrasound examinations will require direct supervision until the resident is able to consistently demonstrate normal anatomy and orientation. Continuing ultrasound examinations performed by the resident should be videotaped, labeled, and reviewed for teaching and quality assurance purposes.

This model curriculum can also serve as a basis for determining training guidelines for board-certified practicing emergency physicians. Physicians who complete 40 hours of continuing medical education (CME) credit in ultrasonography (covering topics that generally follow this outline) and 150 total examinations should be considered trained in emergency medicine ultrasonography.

These recommendations are consistent with those established by other clinical-based specialties. The American Board of Cardiology recommends 3 months of training (or equivalent) in ultrasonography and 120 examinations to achieve the initial level of training.[71] The minimum training recommendations by the Society of OB/Gyn Ultrasonography for a practicing physician with no formal ultrasound experience is either (1) 2 weeks of hands-on instruction, (2) 50 American College of Obstetricians and Gynecologists (A.C.O.G.) CME hours, or (3) 1 week of hands-on training plus 25 A.C.O.G. hours. The American Institute of Ultrasound in Medicine recommends a minimum of 1 month of supervised training and at least 200 examinations for post-residency training in obstetric and gynecologic ultrasound. The German Board of Surgeons requires 300 examinations performed during residency training. It should be pointed out that each of these training guidelines includes many topics not addressed in this model curriculum and not pertinent to emergency medicine.

A broader range of topics could have been covered in the additional uses/issues section. We have chosen to limit the topics to those discussed in the emergency medicine literature or those that are clinically useful. This additional material may be useful for emergency medicine

programs when the interest, clinical material, and educational commitment exists. Further research is needed to determine the benefit and appropriateness of incorporating these techniques into routine emergency medicine practice. This model curriculum may need to be revised and updated as the use of emergency ultrasonography develops.

SUMMARY

A model curriculum for the implementation and training of physicians in emergency medicine ultrasonography is described. Widespread use of limited bedside ultrasonography by emergency physicians will improve diagnostic accuracy and efficiency, increase the quality of care, and prove to be a cost-effective technique for the practice of emergency medicine.

REFERENCES

1. Jehle D, Davis E, Evans T, et al: Emergency department sonography by emergency physicians. Am J Emerg Med 1989;7:605–611.
2. Plummer D, Brunette D, Asinger R, et al: Emergency department echocardiography improves outcome in penetrating cardiac injury. Ann Emerg Med 1992; 21:709–712.
3. Bocka JJ, Overton DT, Hauser A: Electromechanical dissociation in human beings: An echocardiographic evaluation. Ann Emerg Med 1988;17:450–452.
4. Mayron R, Gaudio FE, Plummer D, et al: Echocardiography performed by emergency physicians: Impact on diagnosis and therapy. Ann Emerg Med 1988;17:150–154.
5. Merz RH, Schiller NB: Echocardiography improves emergency room diagnosis. Learning Center Highlights April 1987;15–19.
6. Hauser AM: The emerging role of echocardiography in the emergency department. Ann Emerg Med 1989; 18:1298–1303.
7. Shuman WP, Hastrup W Jr, Kohler TR, et al: Suspected leaking abdominal aortic aneurysm: Use of sonography in the emergency room. Radiology 1988;168:117–119.
8. Kumura A, Otsuka T: Emergency center ultrasonography in the evaluation of hemoperitoneum: A prospective study. J Trauma 1991;31:20–23.
9. Timor-Tritsch I, Greenidge S, Admon D, et al: Emergency room use of transvaginal ultrasonography by obstetrics and gynecology residents. Am J Obstet Gynecol 1992;166:866–872.
10. ACEP Council Resolution on Ultrasound. ACEP Newsletter November 1990.
11. SAEM Ultrasound Position Statement. SAEM Newsletter Summer 1991.
12. Kremkau FW: Diagnostic Ultrasound: Principles, Instruments, and Exercises, 3rd ed. Philadelphia: W. B. Saunders, 1989.
13. Fleischer AC, James AE: Diagnostic Sonography: Principles and Clinical Applications. Philadelphia: W. B. Saunders, 1989.
14. Boswell R: Ultrasonography in Emergency Medicine

Video Program: 301 University Blvd., Emergency Service—Route J73, Galveston, TX 77555-1073.

15. Ultrasound Physics Computer Program. Sonicor, Inc., P.O. Box 347, West Point, PA 19486.

16. Feigenbaum H: Echocardiography, 4th ed. Philadelphia: Lea & Febiger, 1986.

17. Henry WL, Demaria A, Gramiak R, et al: Report of the American Society of Echocardiography, Committee on Nomenclature and Standards in Two-Dimensional Echocardiography. Circulation 1980;62:212–217.

18. Wilson DB, Vacek JL: Echocardiography: Basics for the primary care physician. Postgrad Med 1990;87:191–202.

19. Conrad SA, Byrnes TJ: Diastolic collapse of the left and right ventricles in cardiac tamponade. Am Heart J 1988;115:475–478.

20. Oh JK, Shub C, Miller FA, et al: Role of two-dimensional echocardiography in the emergency room. Echocardiography 1985;2:217–226.

21. Come PC: Echocardiographic recognition of pulmonary arterial disease and determination of its course. Am J Med 1988;84:384–394.

22. Pandian NG, Kusay BS: Use of emergency echocardiography. Cardiology 1989;111–119.

23. Buda A: The role of echocardiography in the evaluation of mechanical complications of acute myocardial infarction. Circulation 1991;I:109–121.

24. Pierard LA, Albert A, Henrard L, et al: Incidence and significance of pericardial effusion in acute myocardial infarction as determined by two-dimensional echocardiography. J Am Coll Cardiol 1986;8:517–520.

25. Schiavone WA, Ghumrawi BK, Catalano DR, et al: The use of echocardiography in the emergency management of non-penetrating traumatic cardiac rupture. Ann Emerg Med 1991;20:1248–1250.

26. Hagen-Ansert SL: Textbook of Diagnostic Ultrasonography, 3rd ed. St. Louis: C. V. Mosby, 1989.

27. Higashi Y, Mizushima A, Matsumoto H: Introduction to Abdominal Ultrasonography. New York: Springer-Verlag, 1991:7–19, 26–33, 156–157.

28. Jeffrey RB: CT and Sonography of the Acute Abdomen. New York: Raven Press, 1989.

29. Marston WA, Ahlquist R, Johnson G, et al: Misdiagnosis of ruptured abdominal aortic aneurysms. J Vasc Surg 1992;16:17–22.

30. Rosenthal SJ, Cox GG, Wetzel LH, et al: Pitfalls and differential diagnosis in biliary sonography. Radiographics 1990;10:285–311.

31. Sinclair D, Wilson S, Toi A, et al: The evaluation of suspected renal colic: Ultrasound scan versus excretory urography. Ann Emerg Med 1989;18:556–559.

32. Rumack CM, Wilson SR, Charboneau JW: Diagnostic Ultrasound. St. Louis: C. V. Mosby Year Book, 1991.

33. Tiling T, Bouillon B, Schmid A, et al: Ultrasound in blunt abdominothoracic trauma. In Border J (ed): Blunt Multiple Trauma: Comprehensive Pathophysiology and Care. New York: Marcel Dekker, 1990:415–433.

34. Filiatrault D, Longer D, Patriquin H, et al: Investigation of childhood blunt abdominal trauma: A practical approach using ultrasound as the initial diagnostic modality. Pediatr Radiol 1987;17:373–379.

35. Callen PW: Ultrasonography in OB/GYN, 2nd ed. Philadelphia: W. B. Saunders, 1988.

36. Timor-Tritsch IE, Rottem S: Transvaginal Sonography, 2nd ed. New York: Elsevier Science Publishing, 1991.

37. Matthews CP, Coulson PB, Wild RA: Serum progesterone levels as an aid in the diagnosis of ectopic pregnancy. Obstet Gynecol 1986;68:390.

38. Stovall TG, Ling FW, Cope BJ, et al: Preventing ruptured ectopic pregnancy with a single serum progesterone. Am J Obstet Gynecol 1989;160:1425–1431.

39. Graham M, Cooperberg PL: Ultrasound diagnosis of interstitial pregnancy: Findings and pitfalls. J Clin Ultrasound 1979;7:433–437.

40. Maliha WE, Gonella P, Degnan EJ: Ruptured interstitial pregnancy presenting as an intrauterine pregnancy by ultrasound. Ann Emerg Med 1991;20:910–912.

41. Rosenberg RD, Williamson MR: Cervical ectopic pregnancy: Avoiding pitfalls in the ultrasonographic diagnosis. J Ultrasound Med 1992;11:365–367.

42. Sherer DM, Abramowicz JS, Thompson HO, et al: Comparison of transabdominal and endovaginal sonographic approaches in the diagnosis of a case of cervical pregnancy successfully treated with Methotrexate. J Ultrasound Med 1991;10:409–411.

43. Abbott J, Emmans LS, Lowenstein SR: Ectopic pregnancy: Ten common pitfalls in diagnosis. Am J Emerg Med 1990;8:515–522.

44. Kurtz AB, Shlansky-Goldberg RD, Choi HY, et al: Detection of retained products of conception following spontaneous abortion in the first trimester. J Ultrasound Med 1991:10:387–395.

45. Pearlman MD. Tintinalli JE, Lorenz RP: Blunt trauma during pregnancy. N Engl J Med 1990;323:1609–1613.

46. Sabia P, Afrookteh A, Touchstone DA, et al: Value of regional wall motion abnormality in the emergency room diagnosis of acute myocardial infarction: A prospective study using two-dimensional echocardiography. Circulation 1991;84:85–92.

47. Peels CH, Visser CA, Funke Kupper AJ, et al: Usefulness of two-dimensional echocardiography for immediate detection of myocardial ischemia in the emergency room. Am J Cardiol 1990;65:687–691.

48. Stiles S: Echo in ER for acute MI could cut needless CCU admissions. Cardiol News 1989;22–27.

49. Oh JK, Miller FA, Shub C, et al: Evaluation of acute chest pain syndromes by two-dimensional echocardiography: Its potential application in the selection of patients for acute reperfusion therapy. Mayo Clin Proc 1987;62:59–66.

50. Goldberger JJ, Hemelman RB, Wolfe CL, et al: Right ventricular infarction: Recognition and assessment of its hemodynamic significance by two-dimensional echocardiography. J Am Soc Echo 1991;4:140–146.

51. Seward JB, Khandheria BK, Oh JK, et al: Transesophageal echocardiography: Technique, anatomic correlations, implementation and clinical applications. Mayo Clin Proc 1988;63:649–680.

52. Shenoy MM, Dhala A, Khanna A: Transesophageal echocardiography in emergency medicine and critical care. Am J Emerg Med 1991;9:580–587.

53. Porembka DT, Hoit BD: Transesophageal echocardiography in the intensive care patient. Crit Care Med 1991;19:826–835.

54. Rooke TW, Martin RP: Lower extremity venous imaging for the echocardiologist. J Am Soc Echo 1990;3:158–169.

55. Marn CS, Bree RL: Advances in pelvic ultrasound: Endovaginal scanning for ectopic gestation and graded compression sonography for appendicitis. Ann Emerg Med 1989;18:1304–1309.

56. Ooms HW, Koumans RK, Ho Kang You PJ, et al: Ultrasonography in the diagnosis of acute appendicitis. Br J Surg 1991;78:315–318.

57. Patten RM, Vincent LM, Wolner-Hanssen P, Thorpe E Jr: Pelvic inflammatory disease: Endovaginal sonography with laparoscopic correlation. J Ultrasound Med 1990;9:681–689.

58. Bulas DI, Ahlstrom PA, Sivit CJ, et al: Pelvic inflammatory disease in the adolescent: Comparison of transabdominal and transvaginal sonographic evaluation. Radiology 1992;183:435–439.

59. Holsbeeck M, Intrasco J: Musculoskeletal Ultrasound. St. Louis: Mosby Year Book, 1991.
60. Schlager D, Sanders AB, Wiggins D, et al: Ultrasound for the detection of foreign bodies. Ann Emerg Med 1991;20:189–191.
61. Gilbert FJ, Campbell RSD, Bayliss AP: The role of ultrasound in the detection of non-radiopaque foreign bodies. Clin Radiol 1990;41:109–112.
62. Crawford R, Matheson AB: Clinical value of ultrasonography in the detection and removal of radiolucent foreign bodies. Injury 1989;20:341–343.
63. Fornage BD, Schernberg FL: Sonographic diagnosis of foreign bodies of the distal extremities. AJR 1986; 147:567–569.
64. Banerjee B, Das RK: Sonographic detection of foreign bodies of the extremities. Br J Radiol 1991;64:107–112.
65. Denys BG, Uretsky BF, Reddy PS, et al: An ultrasound method for safe and rapid venous access. N Engl J Med 1991;324:8.
66. Koski EM, Suhonen M, Mattila MA: Ultrasound-facilitated central venous cannulation. Crit Care Med 1992;20:424–426.
67. Chandraratna PA: Echocardiography and Doppler ultrasound in the evaluation of pericardial disease. Circulation 1991;84:303–310.
68. McGahan JP, Anderson MW, Walter JP: Portable real-time sonographic and needle guidance systems for aspiration and drainage. AJR 1986;147:1241–1246.
69. Cicak N, Matasovic T, Bajraktarevic T: Ultrasonographic guidance of needle placement for shoulder arthrography. J Ultrasound Med 1992;11:135–137.
70. Mayekawa DS, Ralls PW, Kerr RM, et al: Sonographically guided arthrocentesis of the hip. J Ultrasound Med 1989;8:665–666.
71. Prop RL, Winters WL: Clinical competence in adult echocardiography. Circulation 1990;81:2032–2035.

ADDITIONAL RESOURCES

Ultrasound Textbooks

Callen PW: Ultrasonography in OB/GYN, 2nd ed. Philadelphia: W. B. Saunders, 1988.

Feigenbaum H: Echocardiography, 4th ed. Philadelphia: Lea & Febiger, 1986.

Fleischer AC, James AE: Diagnostic Sonography: Principles and Clinical Applications. Philadelphia: W. B. Saunders, 1989.

Hagen-Ansert SL: Textbook of Diagnostic Ultrasonography, 3rd ed. St. Louis: C. V. Mosby, 1989.

Higashi Y, Mizushima A, Matsumoto H: Introduction to Abdominal Ultrasonography. New York: Springer-Verlag, 1991.

Holsbeeck M, Intrasco J: Musculoskeletal Ultrasound. St. Louis: Mosby Year Book, 1991.

Jeffrey RB: CT and Sonography of the Acute Abdomen. New York: Raven Press, 1989.

Kremkau FW: Diagnostic Ultrasound: Principles, Instruments, and Exercises, 3rd ed. Philadelphia: W. B. Saunders, 1989.

Mittelstaedt CA: Abdominal Ultrasound. New York: Churchill Livingstone, 1987.

Rumack CM, Wilson SR, Charboneau JW: Diagnostic Ultrasound. St. Louis: C. V. Mosby Year Book, 1991.

Sarti DA: Diagnostic Ultrasound: Text and Cases, 2nd ed. Chicago: Year Book Medical Publishers, 1987.

Timor-Tritsch IE, Rottem S: Transvaginal Sonography, 2nd ed. New York: Elsevier Science Publishing, 1991.

Educational Videos

Boswell R: Ultrasonography in Emergency Medicine Video Program, 301 University Blvd., Emergency Service—Route J73, Galveston, TX 77555-1073.

Gulfcoast Ultrasound: Introduction to abdominal sonography series: The basics of abdominal sonography, P.O. Box 66700, St. Petersburg Beach, FL 33736; (813) 345–8174.

Gulfcoast Ultrasound: Introduction to adult echocardiography: vol. 1, P.O. Box 66700, St. Petersburg Beach, FL 33736; (813) 345–8174.

Gulfcoast Ultrasound: Introduction to obstetrical ultrasound, P.O. Box 66700, St. Petersburg Beach, FL 33736; (813) 345–8174.

Gulfcoast Ultrasound: Introduction to gynecological ultrasound, P.O. Box 66700, St. Petersburg Beach, FL 33736; (813) 345–8174.

Glossary

A-mode   The type of ultrasound display in which the degree of echogenicity is interpreted as a single point on a vertical axis corresponding to the amplitude and time is displayed on the horizontal axis.

Acoustic shadowing   A phenomenon by which a strong absorber or reflector of sound blocks further passage of ultrasound waves. This creates a dark or anechoic area distal to it. Partial acoustic shadowing results in an area of hypoechogenicity.

Anechoic   Refers to an area where there is no reflection of ultrasound waves, thus appearing dark on the ultrasound screen. The lack of reflections is also referred to as echo-free or sonolucent.

Attenuation   The property by which an ultrasound beam decreases in intensity as it passes through a region. This is caused by absorption, diffraction, interference, reflection, refraction, and scatter.

B-mode   Method of display by which the intensity of reflected ultrasound echoes is depicted by the degree of brightness on the ultrasound screen.

Clean acoustic shadow   One in which there are no reverberation artifacts in the optimal part of the shadow.

Color Doppler   The use of different colors on the Doppler-ultrasound image to indicate different flow velocities.

Coupling medium   The gel or lotion used to ensure good contact between the transducer and the skin surface.

Dirty acoustic shadows   Shadows associated with reverberation artifacts originating at their origin. This is more likely to occur with shadows caused by a gas−tissue interface.

Doppler   Technique that uses ultrasound waves to detect motion of blood within vessels or the heart. The change in frequency of the reflected waves is a function of direction and velocity.

Echo   The reflected ultrasound wave. It is also used as an informal synonym for an ultrasound procedure, particularly of cardiac or vascular structures.

Echocardiogram An ultrasound study of the heart or great vessels.

Echogenic A medium that produces echoes on the ultrasound screen. Usually used in the relative sense; structure A is more echogenic than structure B.

Enhancement An increase in intensity of the reflected ultrasound echoes due to a location distal to an anechoic or relatively hypoechoic structure. The increase in distal echoes is a result of relatively less attenuation of the ultrasound beam as it passes through the proximal structure.

Far gain The degree of amplification used to display the image in the part of the field farthest from the transducer head. It is controlled by the time gain compensator (TGC).

Focal length Distance from the transducer at which the ultrasound beam is most intense. It varies for different transducers and determines at what depth optimum imaging can be obtained.

Gain Measure of the degree of amplification of the signal coming from the transducer.

Gray scale Use of shades of gray to represent amplitude of reflected ultrasound signals.

High resolution (transducer) A probe with a frequency of 7.5 MHz or more.

Hyperechoic A region more reflective of ultrasound waves than another region or structure.

Hypoechoic A region or structure less reflective of ultrasound waves than what it is being compared to.

Linear array transducer (or scanner) A transducer in which many separate piezoelectric elements are set in a linear fashion and are fired sequentially. A rectangular image is produced.

M-mode A one-dimensional ultrasound display where the amplitude is depicted against time; now basically limited to echocardiography.

Mechanical sector scanner Use of a single piezoelectric element or several elements that are moved mechanically rather than electronically. It generates a pie-shaped image.

Megahertz (MHz) Measure of the frequency of ultrasound waves. One MHz equals 10^6 Hz or 1,000,000 cycles per second. Frequencies used in emergency department ultrasound generally range from 3.0 to 7.5 MHz.

Near field That region of the ultrasound display closest to the transducer where the waveforms are unequal. It is followed by the focal zone where the beam width is the narrowest (best imaging). The far-field is just distal to the focal zone and is characterized by increasing beam width.

Piezoelectric effect A phenomenon by which certain substances, particularly quartz and some ceramics, generate electricity upon the application of pressure and conversely generate vibrations upon application of an alternating current. Ultrasound probes use this effect to generate ultrasound waves.

Probe Synonymous with transducer; that piece of ultrasound equipment that transmits and receives ultrasound waves.

Pseudo sludge This artifact can occur when the focal zone is at the center of the gallbladder and the beam is of greater width at the posterior border of the gallbladder. The partial volume effect along the posterior wall results in the appearance of particulate matter or sludge in the gallbladder.

Real-time Type of ultrasound display in which there is no appreciable delay between generation of the ultrasound signal and image formation; sufficient images are generated to allow for the continuous visualization of motion.

Resolution The ability of an ultrasound device to discriminate two closely spaced, reflecting points as separate entities.

Reverberation artifacts Spaced, parallel lines produced when ultrasound signals reflect back and forth between reflecting surfaces.

Scaler Doppler Method to display velocities in a graphic (rather than colorimetric) manner.

Side-lobe artifacts Incorrect superimposition of images produced by reception of ultrasound signals that are not part of the main beam (side lobes).

Sonogram/sonography Synonymous with ultrasound.

Spacer Object or material placed between the transducer and the skin surface in order to achieve a more optimal focal length with a good acoustic window.

Time gain compensator (TGC) The control on an ultrasound device that allows for manipulation of the intensity of the reflected signals in different parts of the ultrasound field. Optimal time gain compensation occurs when the attenuation of signals from the distal field is matched by the amplification of these signals.

Transducer Part of the ultrasound apparatus that transmits and receives ultrasound signals.

Transesophageal echo (TEE) A specialized use of ultrasound utilizing a high-frequency transducer placed in the esophagus for detailed imaging of the heart and great vessels; particularly useful for the detection of aortic dissection.

Index

Note: Page numbers set in *italics* refer to illustrations. Page numbers followed by (t) refer to tables; page numbers followed by *d* refer to definitions of glossary terms.